T0271969

How to Publish in Biological Sciences

How to Publish in Biological Sciences

A Guide for the Uninitiated

John Measey

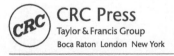

CRC Press
Taylor & Francis Group
Boca Raton London New York

CRC Press is an imprint of the
Taylor & Francis Group, an **informa** business

First edition published 2023
by CRC Press
6000 Broken Sound Parkway NW, Suite 300, Boca Raton, FL 33487-2742

and by CRC Press
4 Park Square, Milton Park, Abingdon, Oxon, OX14 4RN

CRC Press is an imprint of Taylor & Francis Group, LLC

ISBN: 978-1-032-11644-0 (hbk)
ISBN: 978-1-032-11641-9 (pbk)
ISBN: 978-1-003-22088-6 (ebk)

DOI: 10.1201/9781003220886

Typeset in CMR10
by KnowledgeWorks Global Ltd.

To all Early Career Biological Scientists...

May some of your struggles be reduced in size by the contents of this book

Contents

List of Tables

List of Figures

Welcome

Welcome to my guide on how to publish in the Biological Sciences. This guide is pitched at the early career researcher. It is not going to tell you what to write, but to open and examine the black box of scientific publishing, and more broadly explore how this impacts the academic context. My intention is to demystify publication in the Biological Sciences, so that authors become aware of what is happening once they have submitted a manuscript, and how to better interpret the decisions made by colleagues who are reviewing and editing your work.

Publishing has become vital for all academics, such that it is widely recognised that we inhabit a 'publish or perish' academic landscape. For some the process appears effortless, while for others publishing represents a black box leaving them outside in a highly stressful environment. This book is meant to be a guide to those uninitiated members of the academic community, postgraduate students and early career researchers, to bring them up to speed with all the necessary background information on publishing, providing links and references for reading and learning more.

Why read this book

Publishing a paper in an academic journal should simply consist of submitting a publication-worthy manuscript. But having a working knowledge of publishing will enable you to make better decisions about what, where and how to submit manuscripts. This all comes with experience, and in this book, I try to explore the areas of assumed knowledge, and furnish them with explanations pitched at the Early Career Researcher, along with links and citations where you can read more. I explain the many choices that exist for those wishing to submit a manuscript for publication in the Biological Sciences. Where possible, information in this book is tailored for the Biological Sciences, and when this information was not available I used data for the Life Sciences, STEM or science (in that order). I explore the world of publication bias, and how this is evidenced by reviewers and editors. In many cases, Impact Factors, citations and the desire to track the performance of academics has led to unethical practices and exploitation of science and scientists. This guide provides an 'everything you wanted to know about publishing but were afraid to ask' approach for anyone who still feels that submitting a manuscript is like posting it into a black box. This book is written to get you onto an even footing.

What's not in this book

Depending on just how early you are in your career, there is a lot missing from this book that has been provided in another book, *How to Write a PhD in Biological Sciences*[1]. That book concentrates on getting PhD students started writing data chapters, while this book concentrates on publishing manuscripts. Hence, if you want extra information about writing in the Biological Sciences, I would point you to the other book. If you are happy with what you have written, but want help to demystify the publishing process, then this is the right book for you.

Structure of the book

This book is written in four parts:

Part I – Getting your manuscript ready for submission Although you may have already done your research and written your manuscript, getting it ready for publication will require a new set of hurdles for you to jump over. In this section, I discuss what you need to know before entering into the publication arena. What are scientific journals for, and who are the gatekeepers? How does peer review work? The publishing world is at a turning point, and before you start publishing you should be aware of the current reality in Biological Sciences around the currency of citations and how these relate to other metrics such as the Impact Factor and career advancement. You also need to know potential directions for publishing, including the need for transparency in your work, whether or not you should deposit your manuscript as a preprint and who you should invite to be an author. Tactical chapters for Early Career Researchers provide information on how to actively build and maintain a network to facilitate and support your work.

---

[1] www.howtowriteaphd.org

Part II – Submission, reviews and reviewing, revising and resubmitting Sending a paper to a journal is like posting it into a black box where, after some time, you might simply get a rejection and have no idea what has happened. In this section, I take you through the mechanisms of submitting a manuscript from choosing the right journal for your submission, writing a letter to the editor, suggesting reviewers and entering metadata about your manuscript into the editorial management software, all the way to pressing the submit button. I explain how the editorial submission system works, and what you can expect from editors and peer reviewers. I take a practical approach to writing a rebuttal and explain how and why you should expect to revise your manuscript for the editor. The eventual goal of this section is to demystify the entire process between submission and acceptance, and to understand the process from the viewpoint of an author, editor and reviewer.

Part III – Once your paper is published Once your article is accepted, you can celebrate together with your co-authors! You will need to submit the final version of your manuscript, have this type-set and then approve the proofs before a Version of Record appears. At this point, you can start to share your paper, but there are still some key steps that you can take to improve the dissemination of the research to the academic community, to your funders and the public at large. Who is it best to share your research with, and what would be the best form to share it in? In this Part, there are chapters that explain how to write a press release and a popular article on your paper, and how you can improve and monitor its circulation both in academia and in the general media and social media, focussing on those stakeholders who might use your findings.

Part IV – Further challenges in academia The last part of this book discusses the wicked problem posed by current publication models in academia. This Part deals with the growing number of issues driven by a 'publish or perish' culture, and what this means for Early Career Researchers. Special focus is given to the paywall erected by many publishers, Open Access publishing and predatory publishers. I also explain the problems in the current system of biases in peer review, and the confirmation bias in scientific publishing. Instead of just presenting you with problems, this section provides insight into ideas that the academic community has produced in order to get over the current problems. Other important hurdles that you might meet, such as retractions, fraud and bullying, receive in-depth focus.

Why 'A Guide for the Uninitiated'?

Early Career Researchers are within eight years of getting their PhD or within six years of their first academic job. At this time, you will have already experienced the academic life, including publishing, but there will be far more to it than you are aware of. This book considers Early Career Researchers as colleagues who simply lack the experience of a system that has changed in many ways over the last 20 years. To those of you who know the current publishing scene in Biological Sciences, it offers the perspective of where things have come from. I have written this book as I feel that I would have been able to achieve more had I understood more about the publishing process early on in my own career. If I had only had a guide to tell me what it was all about, I could have saved myself so much stress, time and energy. In short, I feel that I was uninitiated, and this is the guide I wish that I had had. So, this guide is my practical attempt to help you; to get you up to speed in the world of academic publishing, specifically in the Biological Sciences. After reading this book, I hope that you will avoid the nightmare world of publishing – of constant effort ending in dead-end rejections that so many academics describe.

Acknowledgements

There are a great many people that I need to thank. First and foremost are the members of my lab, past and present, who have inspired me to put together first the blog posts and then the book. It is because you wanted more that I put this together. This book contains lots of links to blogs and articles written and posted freely on the internet by others who also aim to demystify and help. I thank this greater academic community (especially #academicTwitter) for sharing and inspiring. Thanks go to the many reviewers and editors who have taken their time to improve my writing. I am still learning. Lots of the text in this book has been improved by feedback from my students and postdocs. A special mention must go to my brother, Richard, who has hosted my lab website for more than a decade, and especially for saving blog posts from hacking attacks. Thanks also to Thalassa Matthews, who proofread many of the blog posts after I had published them late at night, so that I could correct them over breakfast in the morning. Graham Alexander, James Baxter-Gilbert, Dan Bolnick, Jack Dougherty, João Fontiela, Thomas Guillemaud, Anthony Herrel, Michael Hochberg, Andrea Hurst, Allan Ellis, Rachael Lammey (CrossRef), Andrea Melotto, Lisa and Mark O'Connell, Ivan Oransky (Retraction Watch), Heather Piwowar (ImpactStory), Claire Riss

(Center for Open Science), Johan Rooryck (cOAltition S), Daniel van Blerk, James Vonesh and Carla Wagener all read or commented on different aspects of the book. Thanks are also due to my colleagues at the Centre for Invasion Biology, the Department of Botany and Zoology, and Stellenbosch University. A special thanks to the librarians who have supported many of my more-extreme rantings about publishers.

John Measey
Cape Town

About the Author

John Measey is an Associate Professor of Biological Sciences at Stellenbosch University. He has authored or co-authored more than 200 peer-reviewed scientific papers and book chapters and five books. He has been the Editor-in-Chief of an ISI journal for nine years, and currently serves as an Associate Editor for four other journals. He has graduated more than 20 postgraduate students, and his blog on writing and publishing in Biological Sciences is read by thousands globally. British born and educated, he lives and works in the beautiful Western Cape, South Africa.

Do you have something to contribute?

This book is written in Bookdown (Xie, 2016) specifically to make it a 'live project' that will be open to anyone who wants to contribute, improve or use as the basis for their own book. The easiest way for readers to contribute content directly is through a GitHub Pull Request[2]. At the repository for this book, you will find Rmd files for each chapter, and as a GitHub user, you can simply edit the Rmd file and submit the changes. If I am happy with the changes proposed, I will merge your content with that of the book and add your name to the Acknowledgements.

One of the amazing potentials for Bookdown books[3] is that all the files for this book are hosted in a repository on Github[4]. You have the opportunity to fork this repository and write your own version for a different discipline, a different language or for a different region of the world. It is also my hope that this guide can grow to become a community of practice for Early Career Researchers in Biological Sciences. It will not be possible to cover every aspect of publishing in Biological Sciences, and it may be that I have missed ones that are very important to you. Equally, parts of what is currently written will become obsolete as new initiatives begin, and old problems are resolved. For

---

[2]https://help.github.com/articles/about-pull-requests/
[3]https://bookdown.org/
[4]https://github.com/johnmeasey/How-to-Publish-in-Biological-Sciences/tree/main

this reason, this guide needs to be a 'living document', and anyone who wants to provide feedback or contribute new sections is more than welcome. Please feel free to open an issue, or make a Pull Request if you spot a typo.

If you haven't already, read the other book

How to Write a PhD in Biological Sciences: A Guide for the Uninitiated by John Measey

Embarking on a PhD is intimidating as, for most students, it will be their first experience working within the academic system. The voyage of discovery is often made very frustrating as much of what goes on in academia is assumed knowledge. Academics accumulate knowledge throughout their careers, but what can be done for those who are uninitiated? What is needed is a guide that postgraduate students can refer to before, during and while making decisions about their time within academia. Note that this is not a rulebook. There are times when the guide will be accurate and others when it will be vague but providing some insight to point you in directions where you can explore more. The intention then is to provide you with a starting point from which you can establish your confidence in the academic writing process and build your own creativity.

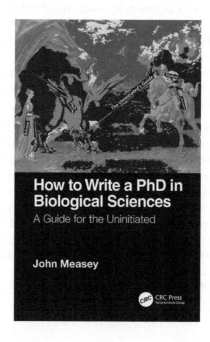

Part I

Getting ready for submission

1

The transition from closed to open

There are a lot of problems in publishing in the Biological Sciences, but it doesn't have to be this way. The aim for this book is firstly to help you navigate the current 'closed' system (while acknowledging that parts are already open), and act as a catalyst towards a more open, transparent and equal system for the future not only of publishing science, but permeating throughout the culture of the scientific project. We have all the tools to make this transition now, and I think that this change will likely come within the time frame of the careers of you as an Early Career Researcher. But as you will see, this change needs to be driven.

While I'm going to pitch the transition from closed to open publishing as a simple process, and as a move from darkness into light, I acknowledge that it might best be defined as a wicked problem. I hope that a lot of these complexities will come out in the book, but acknowledge that a lot will be left unsaid. A large unanswered question is what happens to all the downstream impacts of changing a lucrative academic publishing business that employs tens of thousands of people. I like to think that many of these skilled people, who themselves are not recipients of the large fees acquired by the publishers, would be absorbed into the repurposed institutional libraries. No doubt, there will be casualties. But my belief is that the importance of the scientific project, and the wicked problem we currently face in academic publishing, far outweighs the problems that we will see during the transition.

Throughout this book, I will make reference to the 'scientific project' as a broader philosophical stance in which our studies in Biological Sciences are simply a part (see Measey, 2021). This is a stronger institution without the culture of assumed knowledge and elitism that we see today. I consider movement away from the current model of publishing to be at the heart of this essential institutional transformation.

DOI: 10.1201/9781003220886-1

1.1   Three fundamentals of publishing in Biological Sciences

There are three fundamental concepts that lie at the heart of understanding of current publishing models in the Biological Sciences (Figure 1.1). In themselves, none of them should be particularly influential as they don't relate to your study, how well the study was done, or what your results were. Nevertheless, these three aspects of publishing are key in your understanding of the nuances of publishing, and your understanding will likely make the difference between publishing your work being an obstacle that is occasionally insurmountable, and finding your way with a lot more ease through the process.

1.1.1   Gatekeepers

The journal editor is the kingpin and sits at the centre of this triangle, and has the power, backed by their gatekeeping advisory board and associate editors, to continue the current model, or oversee the change. Editors make decisions, not simply whether to accept or reject your manuscript, but also to implement policies who take their journals in one direction or another. In some models, they are given this power (usually democratically) by the scholarly society that they represent and oversight is granted by an editorial board who mediate in any dispute, but also in theory have influence over the editorial policy. Editors appoint associates who handle many of the manuscripts that are submitted, shuffling them between reviewers and authors until they feel that they are worthy of publication (or not). These associate editors are also responsible for implementing the policies of the editor, the editorial board and the scholarly society. In models where there is only a (for-profit) publisher, the publisher appoints the editor and together they appoint the editorial board. In both models, the editorial board editors and associate editors are thought of as being the gatekeepers to the scholarly integrity that permeates scientific publishing. There is more information on the advisory and editorial boards in Part I.

Gatekeeping takes a lot of time and effort, and there are plenty of places where the current system lacks the transparency that is needed. In theory, there's nothing wrong with this model, were it not for some for-profit publishers that have used the system for their own gain. Instead of the gatekeepers focussing on science, they have become distracted by metrics and hype promoted by publishers. Each of the three facets that surround the gatekeepers in the current publishing model (Figure 1.1) need to be changed to open up the system for a more equitable future, and eliminate the current biases that favour the select few.

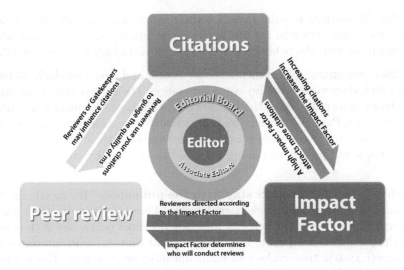

FIGURE 1.1: A schematic for the three fundamentals of publishing in the current Biological Sciences model. Citations, peer review and Impact Factors each have a direct impact on each other and your understanding of each one and how they relate to the other will be pivotal in clarifying your understanding of how to publish your work. At the heart of the process are the gatekeepers: Editorial board, associate editors and the editor.

1.1.2 Is it possible to do without the publishers?

Editors don't have a complete free reign over what to do with their journal. They may be constrained by the publishers, if their journal is run on a for-profit model, or by a contract with a publisher, for most society journals. Journals which are independent of societies and publishers are very rare, but do exist. However they work, editors sit as king-pins of the system. There are examples of editors who have taken all of their associate editors and authors and moved their entire platform to a not-for-profit system. This has also meant changing the name of the journal, as the publisher often owns this. The first example, that I'm aware of, happened in 2015 in the social sciences where the editor of *Lingua* walked away from publishers Elsevier (see Baković, 2017). As Elsevier owned the name, the editor, Johan Rooryck, started a new Open Access journal *Glossa* (www.glossa-journal.org). There was a fight (see Rooryck's website: www.rooryck.org/interaction-with-elsevier), but Rooryck showed that it could be done, and has therefore paved the way for others. Not only did Rooryck show proof of concept, but he formed the Fair Open Access Alliance (www.fairopenaccess.org), who have managed to pull 6 titles away from Elsevier since *Lingua* flipped. It is important to add here that when the gatekeepers leave, the publisher simply approaches new people to take over, and the old journals remain alongside the new. It appears that there is no shortage of academics who are prepared to step into the shoes of editors who part company with the publishers. See what motivates editors in section 3.2.2.

All editors are answerable to their advisory board, and to the scholarly society from which they were (usually) voted into office. The society (often through the editor) signs a deal with the publisher, and this usually runs for a period of 5 years (see Part IV). Society journals usually own their own content and title, and so can decide to leave the publisher whenever their contract expires. It just takes will power, and being prepared to say goodbye to that income stream.

So why do the gatekeepers stay with the publishers? It's mostly smoke and mirrors. Editors and gatekeepers in general are busy people. Their gate-keeping roles are not their primary jobs (for the most part), and if they are then the publishers are paying their wages. What they are most interested in is a smooth system that works with minimum effort on their part. This is what the publishers have established so well, and the principle way in which they will try to persuade gatekeepers to stay with them. Next is the money, which flows from the publishers into the accounts of the societies, with occasional small amounts to editors (and in rare cases associate editors) as expenses. Such perks used to be more substantial, like trips to conferences, hotel stays and wining and dining. But I understand that this is largely gone now. The perceived prestige and professional advancement are discussed in detail later for all gatekeepers. Last is the inertia on the part of gatekeepers to change, as they don't experience the pain of the authors or the libraries that pour money into the publishers. This is a reason why bringing societies into closer contact with institutions is an important step in the process.

1.2   Peer review

Few would argue that peer review is at the heart of publishing in science today. Consequently, there are several chapters in this book concerned with the subject: What is peer review; what to expect from your peer reviewers; how to respond to peer review with a rebuttal; and how to conduct peer review. The last chapter covers problems with peer review and this digs into some of the real biases that occur during peer review, and with the reviewers themselves. Peer review isn't a perfect system, but in order to get the most from it we need to understand the weaknesses, both as authors and as reviewers. Only through this understanding can we reinvent the publishing system. We should not expect to do away with peer review (although this has been suggested many times in the past, and no doubt will be suggested again in the future), but by understanding the the biases that exist we will be able to make sensible choices despite the limitations.

Changes in the peer review system can make the difference between a highly biased system where editors manipulate the content for their own purposes (networks), or a system that is fair and equitable to all.

1.3 Impact Factor

Impact Factor is a simple metric, and as such there is no need for it to be anything more. But the publishers have managed to weaponise Impact Factor to their advantage such that it has become of overriding importance for many publishing in the Biological Sciences today. But it doesn't have to be this way. To make the most of the system, you will need a thorough understanding of the way in which Impact Factor can control other aspects of publishing, and how the behaviour of the editor can have a profound effect on the Impact Factor. A higher Impact Factor results in more submissions, and this in turn will mean that the editor will have more power over the content of their journal.

1.4 Citations

Sitting above peer review and Impact Factor in Figure 1.1 are citations. Compared to the other two parts of this wicked problem, citations seem to be blameless and without the potential biases of the others. However, citations are the units of control for Impact Factor and can be manipulated by both editors and peer reviewers. Metrics driven by citations are also at the heart of many of the problems in today's publishing world.

1.5 Open Science – a vision of the future

In this book, I advocate a vision for a future of Open Science (Figure 1.2). This future is both open and transparent. Future transparency would mean that there is no need for this book, as there will be no hidden agendas or assumed knowledge needed for Early Career Researchers (ECRs). Instead, it will be a 'what you see is what you get' system.

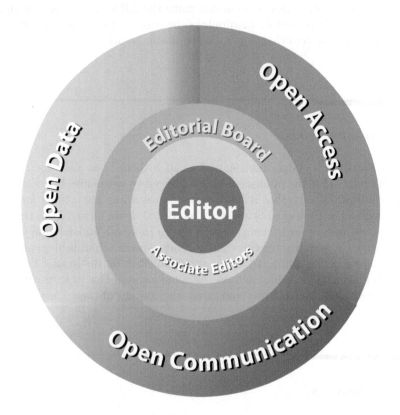

FIGURE 1.2: A simple schematic for an Open Science publishing model. Open science relies on the open nature of publication, communication and data. The gatekeepers still lie at the heart of this model, but are principally involved in ensuring the open and free flow of scientific information. This ideal world is free of the metrics that have dogged research in the past.

The simple schema for Open Science shown in Figure 1.2 is modified from O'Carrroll et al. (2017). The three areas of Open Science start with Open Data, the need to share both data, the code to analyse data, and the details for open source software with which to do the analysis all within open data repositories. The sector on Open Communication replaces the current closed peer review system with an Open framework where all actors are named and any interests declared. These include any journal gatekeepers (if involved). Lastly the publishing of the work is Open Access for other scientists and the public. This includes proposals, preprints, reviews and published articles.

At the heart of Open Science publishing is ownership of the content. Like many aspects of changing the model from closed to open, implementation of the Rights Retention Strategy (see Janicke Hinchliffe, 2021), through mechanisms such as CC-BY[1], is available today. This is something that you, as an author, should insist on anywhere you publish. If the journal refuses, then **think about what are they saying to you.**

In my opinion, the Open Science framework (osf.io) is incompatible with the for-profit scientific publishing model that drives the current model (Figure 1.1). I hope that the transition from Figure 1.1 to Figure 1.2 will be swift, and happen within your career. However, the actors at play in this system are not neutral, and need both bottom-up challenges (from yourselves as ECRs) as well as top-down pressure (especially from large funding agencies). We should acknowledge that changing our research environment within science is not an immediate process, but requires a suite of cultural changes (Figure 1.3), that will start with early adopters and ultimately end with regulated policy (Nosek, 2019). These changes will be as exciting as they are challenging, and I hope that the contents of this book will equip you to participate fully.

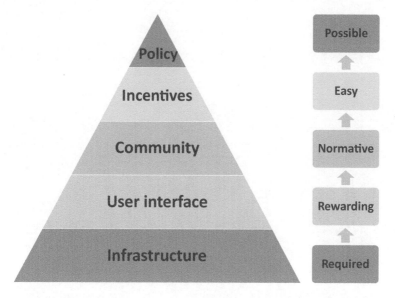

FIGURE 1.3: Changing the prevailing culture in science will take time and effort but is currently possible. This book attempts to provide information about how a change towards Open Science is currently both possible and easy (bottom), but requires widespread adoption among the Biological Sciences community in order to make it normative and rewarding (middle), until we reach ubiquity through policy (top). (Redrawn from Nosek, 2019).

---

[1]https://creativecommons.org/licenses/by/4.0/

2

What is a scientific journal for?

It's worth reflecting on why we have scientific journals, and what they are for. Primarily journals are a means of communication for the academic community. The academic community here should be regarded in the broadest of interpretations. For example, some journals also serve to disseminate research to those who draw-up and implement policy. Others are aimed at managers who want to base their actions on scientific findings. The direction and inclusivity of the audience is pivotal in both what and how we write.

- Journals record and disseminate the findings of individuals and teams of academics from all over the world.
- By having a date when they are published, together with the names of the authors, they record primacy; that is who came up with the finding or idea first. Also see important arguments against the need for primacy (Casadevall and Fang, 2012).
- They attempt to register legitimacy by collating and integrating comments and concerns through peer review.
- Lastly, they archive these findings so that in future people can build on the work.

There are so many scientists in the world publishing so many papers that it's not possible for all scientists to read everything. Today annual growth in scientific papers is 5.1%, equivalent to a doubling time of 13.8 years (Bornmann et al., 2020; see also Part IV). Contrast this with the early days when there were only two journals and they constituted all that was published at the time. Over time a natural hierarchical system of what scientists will read has developed. This is reflected in citations, and the simplest measure of journals is something called the Impact Factor.

It has been said that 'authorship' is a relatively modern concept, emerging from the empiricism of England's middle-ages (see Cronin, 2001). In our recent history, it is considered to be important for individuals to record who thought of what and when. From these authors, we give societal 'author-ity'. This gives credit where it's due. In the big scheme of things of course it's not important who did what. We know from historical examples like natural selection that Darwin and Wallace had very similar thoughts that were a product of many people who were thinking about these ideas at the time. Although certain authors may be 'ahead of their time', the majority of thoughts and ideas that come around today are a product of their time. However, for individuals and their institutions it can be important to claim credit as this may translate into some monetary value (e.g. with patents), or a prestige value. The regulated system of taxonomy puts a lot of importance on the priority of who described what and when.

The system of editors and peer reviewers determining whether or not a manuscript possesses sufficient merit to be published is regularly regarded as the gold standard in science (Mayden, 2012). As you will discover, it is often a very high bar to achieve. Of course both editors and peer reviewers are human and so the system is not perfect. We'll talk more about peer review in the next chapter.

Archiving the findings of scientists is perhaps one of the most important roles of publishers that we should be most concerned about. In my career, I have seen the changes from strictly paper dissemination of scientific findings, as it was for the past 350 years, to primarily electronic findings many of which are never printed by the majority of readers. We should be concerned about how long these records will last. If you have never thought about the longevity of data storage, then this is something that you should give some thought to. We all need to change our perspectives on long-term thinking as this impacts almost every societal function (see the Long Now Foundation longnow.org).

3

What is peer review?

Peer review is often considered to be the 'gold standard' of science (Mayden, 2012). Manuscripts that have passed peer review are regularly considered to have been scrutinised to the highest level. If one's peers in the scientific community consider that a manuscript is worthy of publication, then it meets the high standards of peer review. In theory, the review of peers acts as the guardian to all that is good in science, and excludes all that is bad. A lot has been written about peer review (>23,000 articles!), and there's plenty more to read out there (Eve et al., 2021).

While the views in the above paragraph are generally held, there is also a universal acknowledgement that there are a lot of problems with peer review. That this has been widely acknowledged is probably an understatement, as most people who have experienced it would likely already know. These problems will be addressed in another chapter in the last Part of this book. The myriad of failures means that peer review shouldn't ever be exulted as the 'gold standard' touted by many publishers. Peer review does provide a filter of sorts, with the result being better considered as a 'silver standard'.

But peer review is here to stay and will remain as a fundamental aspect of publishing, and so there are several chapters in this book that are dedicated to different aspects. In this chapter, I attempt to explain what peer review is. Elsewhere there are descriptions:

- what to expect from peer reviewers
- how to respond to peer review
- how to conduct peer review
- problems with peer review

This chapter provides an overview of the topic, but you may need to refer to the other chapters first depending on what your current need is.

DOI: 10.1201/9781003220886-3

3.1   History of peer review

The history of peer review is surprisingly modern. We know that journals
themselves only date back to the 17th century (see chapter in Part IV). These
journals included a form of peer review in that letters concerning studies could
be published, along with comments made at presentations. However, the type
of systematic enforced peer review described in this book is very recent (Eve
et al., 2021). The journal *Nature* for example only started systematic peer
review for its articles in 1973, and mainstream editor led peer review only
really started in the late 1940s (see Tennant, 2017). Typical society journals
have followed a similar form of evolution from newsletters to scholarly journals
(e.g., Measey, 2011).

3.1.1   How high is the peer review bar?

It is difficult to emphasise how high the peer review bar is. When your
manuscript is scrutinised by your peers, it is very rare (practically unheard of in
the careers of most researchers) that it will get accepted without modifications.
This is because the experience of academics tends to be so wide, and vary so
much from individual to individual, that it is almost impossible to predict
what a peer reviewer will see when they read your manuscript.

You should expect that your manuscript will not receive an easy ride through
peer review. But you should also expect that it will be improved. As we will
see later, this improvement might not be immediately obvious to you when
you first read the comments.

It is also important to note that as the author, you are the net beneficiary of
the peer review process, and that once you press the submit button (free for
the vast majority of us, but see part IV), a cascade of events happen, all of
which are done in the name of you and your submission. It stands to reason
then that you should be sure that your manuscript is as ready as it can be for
submission.

3.2   Who are your peers?

Essentially the peers in peer review are people that editors find and persuade
to conduct the peer review. It can be difficult to find people to conduct a peer

review. Although only two or three reviews are needed sometimes as many as 20 or 30 individuals can be approached. Perry et al. (2012) lamented on the increasing difficulty in persuading colleagues to conduct peer review of manuscripts.

While your 'peer' might sound like someone who is in an equivalent position to you, this may not be the case. If you are junior, your peer reviewers may be very senior. Equally, senior authors may have peer reviewers that may be very junior. Does this make a difference? For some people it might, especially when they know the other party and assign some level of competence associated with their seniority. Of course, both junior and senior researchers are capable of getting points in peer review wrong, just as both are also capable of providing insightful feedback. The editors are those in the hotseat about what it all means.

Professionals: Peer reviewers are normally professionals. Academics, postdocs or postgraduate students. Occasionally there are specialist amateurs who have very high academic standards and who can be contacted to conduct peer review. For journals with a special remit, industry professionals may be approached to provide feedback on applied aspects of manuscripts.

Scholars: Peer reviewers should be familiar with the subject area to a good level of scholarly achievement. Undergraduates and many postgraduate students would not be considered eligible by many editors as peer reviewers. Personally I found that many PhD students, especially those in their final stages of studying are very good peer reviewers.

Specialists: Peer reviewers should be specialists to some degree of the area on which the manuscript is based. Often it's not possible to be a specialist in every area of a manuscript. But in the case where you are not proficient it is important to inform the editor.

3.2.1 The role of the editor

The editor has an important role to play:

- To assess your submission
  - Does it align with the journal?
  - Is it sound enough to send to peer review?
  - Whether to use a specialist associate editor
- To choose the peer reviewers
  - Without potential conflicts of interest
  - Who can cover the content of the manuscript
  - Who agree to doing the review within the prescribed time-frame
- To assess the reviews of the reviewers
  - Mitigate for potential bias in the reviews

– Judge what is in the manuscript against what reviewers have found
– Determine whether sufficient merit remains in order to undergo a decision (including more peer review)

- Write the decision: When you bear in mind that the decision is likely to involve some arbitration between different reviewer opinions, and to direct the authors about what changes need to be made to a manuscript in order to make it acceptable, the decision is not a simple exercise. Making an editorial decision will require careful reading of the manuscript, the reviewers' comments, as well as looking past potential biases of reviewers.

3.2.2   Who are the Gatekeepers (Advisory and Editorial Boards)?

The Advisory Board (sometimes referred to confusingly as the Editorial Board) together with the editor and associate editors, make up the gatekeepers of scientific knowledge. Through their combined influence, they determine what knowledge is published by screening submissions and allowing only a proportion of them to be published. The advisory board are invited academics who are often considered to be leaders in the field relating to the journal subject area, and are invited to join by the editor and/or the society. In theory, they are ambassadors for the journal, encouraging authors to submit their manuscripts (e.g. following talks at conferences), identifying new topics for editorials and special issues, and generally supporting the editor and associate editors. The Advisory Board are also there in the case of dispute (especially between authors and editors), or for complaints coming from third parties (against editors or published articles). In general, most issues involving a journal are dealt with by the editor. Only in exceptional circumstances is the Advisory Board consulted. Practically, the role of the Editorial Board is largely passive, and hence many think of the gatekeepers as being only the editor and associate editors.

Here, I refer to the editor and associate editors collectively as the '**Editorial Board**'.

The editorial board are said to support orthodox views in their fields and could be thought of as representing the 'establishment' (Crane, 1967). The argument continues that like supports like, and that editorial boards in science tend to be composed of white men at US universities. One real problem with gatekeepers is their lack of diversity (Potvin et al., 2018). In a study of 250 science journals, only one country on the African continent had gatekeepers represented at 0.16%, while the USA had 53.87% of the gatekeepers (Braun and Dióspatonyi, 2005). Increasing the geographic diversity of the editorial board leads to an increase in the diversity of the authors (Demeter, 2018; Goyanes and Demeter, 2020; Potvin et al., 2018), something as biologists we can all appreciate a real need for.

Editors, sometimes referred to as editors-in-chief (presumably to distinguish them from associate editors) are usually alone in their position at journals. Increasingly, journals with large numbers of submissions have joint editors-in-chief, or even another tier of editorial oversight under the editor-in-chief. The major part of their job is screening the submissions to the journal and assigning the most appropriate associate editor. In most journal models, the editor-in-chief reviews the information provided by the associate editor and make a final decision on whether or not a manuscript is accepted to the journal (see Figure 15.1 later in this book). Their gatekeeping role comes with the many decisions that they have influence over, for example what kinds of articles they will accept, the decision to amend the description of the journal on the website, which will impact how you choose the journal you submit your manuscript to. This is the reason why you are always advised to look at the current content of your journal choice. There is also the important role that the editor takes when things go wrong, which can be very time consuming.

Associate Editors are most likely to be tenure-track faculty in a US research intensive university, according to an illuminating study by Kelsey Poulson-Ellestad and colleagues (2020). Most are within 10 years of earning their PhD, and are therefore still Early Career Researchers, and have published ~20 papers and conducted >50 reviews. Rewards include a better understanding of the publication system, improved communication skills, keeping current in the journal area and giving back to the scientific community. Most of the costs involve time around finding reviewers, reading manuscripts and making difficult decisions, especially around conflicting peer review comments. But editing takes time, and can be burdensome in this respect especially for Early Career Researchers who have so much else on their plate. The advice of many Associate Editors in the study was for others not to take on editing unless they are sure that they can commit enough time (Poulson-Ellestad et al., 2020). Gender equality in Associate Editors of ecological journals has been improving over time, as has the gender equality of reviewers (Fox et al., 2019), although other surveys have found huge disparity of only 16% of subject editors being women in 10 environmental biology and natural resource management journals (Cho et al., 2014). However, women are more likely to refuse an invitation to become an Associate Editor (Fox et al., 2019). The gender imbalance in gatekeepers is indicative of the general imbalance across STEM subjects.

All of the processes in one round of peer review need to be worked around the editor's existing job, professional and research commitments (i.e. the day job), and their home life. The motivations for shouldering this additional work-load will be as individual as there are people in these roles. However, I have summarised some of the acknowledged motivations in Table 3.1.

TABLE 3.1: What are the main motivations for the various gatekeepers? In this table, I summarise what I consider to be the main motivations of the different types of gatekeepers and reviewers of a typical Biological Sciences journal.

Motivation	Editors	Associate editors	Board member	Reviewers
The prestige associated with the journal	X	X	X	-
Increasing their professional network	X	X	-	X
Increase their soft power	X	X	X	X
Participate in the production of knowledge	X	X	-	X
Give back to a system from which you've benefited	X	X	-	X
Part of obtaining tenure	-	X	-	X
Editors-in-Chief are usually selected from among the ranks of the Associate Editors	-	X	-	-
A better understanding of the publication system	-	X	-	-
Keeping current in the journal area	X	X	-	X
Prestige of having your name listed on the journal website	X	X	X	-
An opportunity to use soft power at conferences and other meetings	X	X	X	-
Recognition of being influential in your field	X	X	X	-
Another lever to use in arguing for promotion	X	X	X	-
Complimentary access to the journal	-	-	X	-

3.3   Reviewer models

Reviewers themselves come in different flavours that are (mostly) predetermined by the journal regulations.

3.3.1 Blind reviewers

Blind reviewers know who the authors are, but are anonymous to the author, but known to the editor. This can be considered the 'standard model' in peer review. There are plenty of problems with this model as reviewers may use their anonymity to hide their biases and are even known to become abusive. Although reviewers may be anonymous, sometimes communities are so small that authors might guess who these people are, simply by their comments and suggestions. Although this is the most common type of review format, it is the least recommended. If you feel that there may be potential reviewers who bear a grudge to your laboratory, your institution or your work, then it may be better to avoid this kind of review system.

3.3.2 Double blind reviewers

Double blind reviewers do not know who the authors are, and are anonymous to the author, but known to the editor. The double blind model was conceived to remove some of the potential biases (particularly around gender, nationality and race) that might come about through the identification of the authors and their addresses. Again, it has been mooted, and it is also my experience, that in a small community one tends to know who authors and reviewers are simply by the subject of the manuscript and the comments (see also Eve et al., 2021). However, even when groups can be identified, it is not always possible to determine the author or author combination, and so biases around gender and race may still be avoided with this model.

3.3.3 Triple blind reviewers

In theory, it is possible for the editor, after having chosen the reviewers, to be blinded from their identity once they submit their review. This may prevent the editor putting more importance to a more senior reviewer, and ignoring more junior viewpoints.

3.3.4 Open reviewers

Open reviewers know who the authors are, and are known by the authors and editor. Note that this is a simplification of a complex set of potential openness. For a thorough discussion see Ross-Hellauer (2017). The open reviewer model does encourage good behaviour (or the avoidance of some of the worst problems) on the part of reviewers. However, reviewers remain brutally direct even when they are named, such that even open comments may be construed as bruising by the authors (Eve et al., 2021).

3.3.5   Public reviewers

Public reviewers know who the authors are, and are known by the authors and editor, and their names (and often their reviews) are made available to the public. This model is relatively recent, and comes along with the possibility of making the reviews with their own DOIs (digital object identifiers) available along with the accepted manuscript. It is worth noting that, to date, reviews for manuscripts that are rejected do not get posted using this or any other current publishing model. It does exist in the world of preprints. Public reviews contribute towards Open Science through Open Communication.

This could be considered the most transparent system for any journal. It has also been called Open Evaluation (OE) by Kriegeskorte et al. (2012). *PeerJ* and *eLife* are among a very small handful of journals that have tried to instigate this model. Nevertheless it can be very difficult to find reviewers who are prepared to reveal their names to the authors. A study that compared *PeerJ* publications in which reviews were made public, compared to those that authors chose to keep closed, suggested that the subsequent number of citations increased by a third for open reviews (Zong et al., 2020). It is only possible to speculate about why this might be. The decision at *PeerJ* to open reviews is made first by reviewers (who opt not to be anonymous), and then by authors (who opt to open reviews). In studies where both groups co-operate, we might hope that this results in a higher quality product. Indeed, public reviews tend to be longer, although positive comments are more frequent in closed reviews (Bornmann et al., 2012). It is equally possible that authors who choose to open their peer review are more progressive and active within research (leading to more citations).

3.4   Learn more about peer review by doing it

As an early career researcher, you may well be asked to conduct peer review of an article in your specialist field. If you have never been asked, then tell your mentor to recommend you. Usually when they turn down an opportunity to conduct peer review, they have an opportunity to name someone else. If you have told them that you want some manuscripts to review, it should be straightforward for them to add your name when appropriate.

Another option is to volunteer to conduct peer review for an independent peer review site, like Review Commons (www.reviewcommons.org) or Peerage of Science (www.peerageofscience.org). Here you can register your interest and then take your pick of articles that get submitted. A nice aspect is that Review Commons have Referee Cross-commenting, so that you get to see the other reviewer comments and make additional comments on these as you see fit. Review Commons and Peerage of Science are both excellent platforms on which to get some experience with reviewing.

Similarly, you could post your reviews of preprints online. You might be shy to do this at first, so consider sitting with a lab mate and doing a review together. You can always ask your mentor to take a look at your review if you are unsure whether or not it should be posted publicly.

When you register in the editorial manager software for journals that you submit to, there is often an option to state what areas of your field you are particularly specialised in, and whether or not you are interested in conducting peer review in these areas. This is also worth doing if you want to generate requests for conducting peer review.

Another way of getting noticed is to sign up to society training programmes for peer review. These might happen at conferences, or could be through web-based courses. Although it should be noted that such courses may have little impact to improve your peer review (Schroter et al., 2004), you will certainly gain more insight. You will need to register to conduct such training, with the result (sometimes) that your name will be entered into the editorial management software, together with your trained status. Some courses actually have 'live' mentors who read through and critique reviews that you conduct. All of these are a good idea, but be sure to check out the time commitment required before you start.

Good reviews get noticed by editors, and it is a good way of increasing your network through soft power.

We will look in more detail about how to conduct peer review later in this book.

3.4.1 What do peer reviewers get out of participation?

Table 3.1 suggests that reviewers receive the least out of the system for their efforts. Having simplified this in the table, there are lots of exceptions, and certain journals do provide incentives for reviewers, including free access to their content. Doing a good job of peer review will generate soft power if you renounce your anonymity. Doing this for a journal where your name is displayed alongside the article will help increase your profile.

Note that what reviewers get out of participating in peer review is almost identical to editors (see Table 3.1). Editors benefit at a higher level, mostly as their names are seen more often by more people, but with the drawback that they do a lot more work than the peer reviewer.

I have heard some members of the community claim that they will continue to accept peer review requests until these cover what they are demanding of the community (i.e. reviews offered per year = submissions per year x ~2.5). Although this sounds very fair, I would suggest that the reality is more subtle. You shouldn't be accepting to conduct peer reviews for articles where you feel that you lack specialist knowledge. Neither should you be conducting peer review when you feel that you have a conflict of interest.

If you do have to turn down the invitation of peer review, then do it as soon as possible, and try to suggest someone else that you think could do it.

4

Transparency in publishing

The need for transparency in science stems from the fact that most civic societies are making the majority of their decisions based on evidence coming through the guidance of science. If scientific evidence is at the heart of decision making, then the collection of this evidence must be transparent to those who make resulting policies, together with those who challenge them in a democracy. Moreover, as public funded scientists, we should be setting a community standard of transparency for the rest of society to follow. Publishing of science is currently in transition to address the wicked problem, and it is vital that the scientific community leads the way forward, and that we are not led by for-profit publishers. One of the ways to achieve transparency is through preregistration of your research project to avoid confirmation bias. This bias is, in part, a product of commercial publishers and the metrics they promote. In order to make this effective, we need the gatekeepers of our journals to support the preregistration of research hypotheses and methods. Right now, journals should be openly advocating and encouraging preregistration with a plan to transition their journal in future to a system embracing rigour, reproducibility and transparency (RRT: Valdez et al., 2020). However, many editors are resisting this move as they feel that there is no support from the community. This may well be the case, but inequalities in science, and particularly in publishing, mean that editors can either be instruments of change or at the heart of inequality in publishing (see Part IV and Figure 1.1). Either our editors will lead us towards transparency, or we as a community simply need to demand that they change their practices. Currently, editors are responding to calls for transparency by making small steps (e.g. asking for open coding: Powers and Hampton, 2019), rather than adopting transparency wholesale through the badge system set up by Kidwell et al. (2016).

4.1 Removing the prejudice around confirmatory bias

Confirmatory bias is the phenomenon increasingly seen in science that most studies published accept the alternative hypothesis, even though this is the least likely outcome of any experiment. Confirmation bias happens in publishing as editors prefer to accept papers that have a positive outcome. It has been suggested that this leads to a culture of 'bad science', and even fraud. One convincing set of evidence of confirmation bias is the decline of null results over time (Fanelli, 2012).

4.1.1 Accepting the alternative hypothesis

At the outset of our scientific research we pose a hypothesis with the expectation that we will be able to accept or reject our null hypothesis. We often think of rejecting the null hypothesis as the only result that we are interested in, but if we only ever reported these results we would not be responsible in moving our field forward. That is, in a world where we only report significant results (i.e. reject the null hypothesis) we would necessarily keep repeating experiments where the null hypothesis is accepted, because there would never be the evidence that the hypothesis had been previously tested in the literature. This is actually practised by the majority of scientific journals who won't consider a null result, and results in 'Publication Bias'. It's easy to see why this is a bad policy, but it is the prevailing culture in scientific publishing.

If journals only publish manuscripts that reject the null hypothesis (*cf* Franco et al., 2014), researchers are more likely to mine their data for positive results (P hacking), or re-write their hypothesis in order to reject the null (HARKing) (Measey, 2021). Deceptive practices such as P hacking, HARKing and salami-slicing are not in the interests of any journals, or the scientific project in general (Ioannidis, 2005; Nissen et al., 2016; Forstmeier et al., 2017; Measey, 2021).

4.1.2 Inadvertent bias

Positive results don't only come from deliberate manipulation of results. As humans we are predisposed towards positive results (Nuzzo, 2015), and there are plenty of reasons why researchers might inadvertently reach a false positive outcome (Type I error). Forstmeier et al. (2017) draw attention to cryptic multiple tests during stepwise model simplification, and the two types of researcher degrees of freedom (*sensu* Simmons et al., 2011): stopping rules and flexibility in analysis.

Cryptic multiple tests during stepwise model simplification relates to the way in which adding predictors to models inflates the total number of models to test, making it necessary to adjust alpha accordingly (for repeated tests). However, Forstmeier and Schielzeth (2017) report that even with Bonferroni adjusted alpha levels, they found using random data that models with one significant effect happen around 70% of the time. The only way to keep this under control is to use sufficient sample sizes to maintain the power to distinguish between true positives and false positives. A handy rule of thumb from Field (2013) is that sample size needs to be eight times the number of model predictors plus 50. Better would be to run a power analysis on your study design, and to critically reassess your predictors to eliminate as many as you can before you begin your study.

Researcher degrees of freedom is the way that Simmons et al. (2011) described ways in which researchers may inadvertently increase their chances of getting false positive results during analysis. The first is simply the way in which researchers decide to stop collecting data. Clearly, if preliminary collections showed a trend, but not a significant result, then collecting more data sounds like a good idea. However, as the collection of data is not independent (when the first set is kept) then the first test is not independent of the second, and so the chance of getting a Type I error is cumulative. Even if multiple datasets are collected, those that are insignificant should also be considered and reported in order to get an unbiased estimate. The second major way in which analyses can turn out with false positives is through potentially infinite flexibility in analyses. There are lots of ways to analyse your data and given enough trials, it is quite likely that you'll find one that gives you significant results. Moreover, on the road to conducting the test, there are many options that can change the outcome of the analysis:

- Inclusion or exclusion of an outlier
- Inclusion or exclusion of a covariate
- Transforming dependent variables
- Inclusion or exclusion of baseline measures
- Controlling for sex (or another variable) as a fixed effect
- Excluding individuals with incomplete datasets

The potential list of ways in which the outcome of your analysis could change quickly grows as the number of ways in which you could analyse the data also grows. But don't despair. Transparent help is at hand.

4.1.3   Novel research

One criterion for publication in many journals is that the research should be novel. This is increasingly practiced by journal editors as you move up the Impact Factor levels. Novelty sells (just think of the meaning of 'new' in newspaper), and that's the basis for selling novel stories from higher Impact Factor journals. The perils of testing increasingly unlikely hypotheses, and how this inflates Type II errors as well as increasing the proportion of Type I errors, are widely acknowledged (Forstmeier et al., 2017; Measey, 2021). Novelty also stifles repeatability. If we can never repeat studies in science, then a fundamental tenet of the methodology is repressed. Reproducibility in science has received a lot of attention recently, as attempts to reproduce the results of highly cited research have failed (e.g. Lithgow et al., 2017). This has been followed by general outrage among scientists that things should change (Anderson et al., 2007; Munafò et al., 2017), including a majority of those in Biological Sciences (Baker, 2016). The irony that these reports and requests are published in exactly the journals that will refuse to publish research that seeks to repeat work (is not novel) is clearly lost on the editors. However, more nuanced views are also coming forward to actively introduce variable conditions and sampling of biological variation into the study design to more fully represent the nature of biological variation making studies more likely to be replicated (Voelkl et al., 2020).

4.2 Introducing transparency in peer review

The way in which editors choose and interpret reviewers can either reinforce their own prejudices, or help to make publication more open and transparent for everyone. A first step is moving from double-blind review to triple-blind where editors cannot make decisions with prejudice towards certain reviewers. Next is the need for public reviews with DOIs that allow open assessment of what reviews contained. For more details about problems in peer review, see Part IV.

In order to change this culture to a more transparent selection of scientific studies for publishing, we need journals to sign up to be transparent. Sadly, when most journals are approached, the editors either ignore the email or make an excuse about why it is not possible (Mellor et al., 2019). Of course, some journals have adopted the road to transparency, and we should be encouraged by the fact that they still exist, and that we can build on these initial front runners. In addition, there are a growing number of excellent frameworks that are pointing the way forward (e.g. Macleod et al., 2021). This is a cultural change that we can expect will take time (Figure 1.3).

4.2.1 Moving towards Open Science

Taking out the profiteering from publishers will take a more concerted approach. But the reality is that we have only ourselves to blame. Biological scientists do not challenge the publishing model because we are used to getting all of the 'frills' associated with it. We are used to the prestige that is afforded to the gatekeepers, and for contributors and readers this includes the designer layout, custom websites and editorial management systems and now increasingly the use of free tools like Mendeley, Overleaf, Peerwith and Authorea. Indeed, these and other tools can be used as spyware to capture data from individual academics and sell it (see Brembs et al., 2021). Instead I suggest using not-for-profit repositories and Open Source Tools (Kramer and Bosman, 2016). An excellent way to learn and implement the use of these tools is to form an Open Science Community in your institution (Armeni et al., 2021). There you can learn more from your peers about which tools are best used in your area and with your institutional resources, and help spread the word of the need to move towards Open Science among your colleagues.

The reality is that we really don't need any of these frills. An entire workflow using Open Source Tools is available, and it is up to us to make this convenient for our own use. If we cared more about our science and less about so-called prestige, we'd all be better off. Mathematicians and physicists are way ahead of biologists. Given that they've shown the way, it's simply up to us to embrace openness and transparency.

5

What can you publish?

As you become more familiar with the academic literature, you will quickly realise that actually you can publish just about anything. In this part of the book I'm going to talk about some of the most common articles that you can get published. But don't feel constrained by what you see here. When it comes to publishing you're only constrained by your imagination.

As an early career researcher, you will have a body of work from your thesis that you may have already published, or be in the process of publishing. These likely contain a number of data chapters that will be published as a series of papers in scientific journals. However, it's worth reflecting here about what it is possible to publish and how this might complement your existing and future publications, as well as increasing your publication portfolio with which to further your career. Although publishing is not the only way to do this, having more publications is likely to increase your visibility in your community, as well as giving you more practice in academic writing.

5.1 Standard articles

You should already be familiar with the concept of publishing standard articles and you may already have a number of these published both as a first author and as a co-author. As an Early Career Researcher, you should consider what and how you publish. For example, you should consider whether or not publishing more articles is always the right strategy for you. You will find a chapter that discusses this concept in detail in Part IV. In particular, you should be aware of the concept of salami-slicing a standard article into two or more different papers.

DOI: 10.1201/9781003220886-5

5.2   Reviews

When considering the way in which citations work, one of the things that you should notice is that reviews and in particular meta-analyses are cited many more times than most individual papers. Perhaps more importantly, they give you a novel perspective on your own research area, and can help direct your own work into more relevant areas. For this reason one of the best things you can do is an early career researcher is to author a review on the topic of (or around) your thesis, or even better a meta-analysis.

The importance of a timely and much used review can be seen in a lot of citation maps such as in Figure 5.1. In this example, Ellender & Weyl (2014) was the first comprehensive review that sums the knowledge to that date on invasive fishes in South Africa, and so was cited more times than anyone who published anything on invasive fish species in the country thereafter. Because this subject was the focus of a lot of research that happened in the area, you can see that it would logically sit at the centre of this subdiscipline. If you are unsure about whether or not a review is needed in your subdiscipline, then constructing a citation network based on the key-words in your subdicipline, such as that in Figure 5.1, might well be useful.

5.3   Commentaries or opinion pieces

Your opinion is important, or at least as important as anyone else's. Critical reading is a very important part of science and something that you should maintain throughout your career. From time to time you will come across articles and papers that you know are wrong, or fail to represent sufficient balance. Many journals will accept commentaries or opinion pieces based on articles that they have already published. This is an opportunity for you to make a correction to something that's already published in the literature. Please know that here we are not talking about anything you think might be fraudulent; for that there is another process.

There are several things worth considering before putting pen to paper on your commentary and sending it to the editor.

- If the people that wrote the article are in your network or in a network close to yours then consider approaching them first about what you see as their error. You may end up getting along with them much better when you seek a solution together than writing something that antagonises them. Even if they aren't in your network you may find a way to increase the influence of your network through soft power instead of with a commentary.

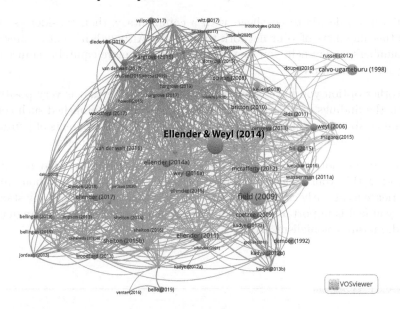

FIGURE 5.1: A timely review can be at the heart of a citation network, such as this one on 'Invasive fish' AND 'South Africa'. In this citation network, you can see that the best cited paper (largest circle – green and centre) is a review by Ellender & Weyl (2014). It has good connections with all of the three subject areas of this citation network, and although it was published in 2014, by 2021 it had been cited 111 times. Drawn with VOSviewer (van Eck and Waltman, 2010).

- A commentary should never be an *ad hominem* attack. Never comment on the authors, only the content.
- Check with your mentor or another colleague that your interpretation of their error is correct and that pointing this out will have some value. Always try to do more than just say: 'no it isn't'. Many journals won't be interested in a commentary that does nothing more than show an error. If possible try and include some original data or some original analyses in your response.
- Remember that your commentary will likely be sent immediately to the authors that you're commenting on before it is accepted by the editor. This means that they will also get a chance to comment on your commentary. However you will not get a chance to look at their comment.
- Have a look through instances of where this has happened in the literature in your field. If you can talk to the people involved, try to find out whether things worked out positively for them. Although I do not want to say that you shouldn't do this, you should know that what you're doing is not going to backfire on you especially as an Early Career Researcher.

- If you do decide to go ahead with a commentary, then consider asking other members of your network to join you. Although it's not a game of numbers it may help you to gauge a better and more equitable stance on your commentary.

The other option you have is publishing a commentary that is very positive about the findings of a particular paper. Some journals published such commentaries about the contents of their journal as well as the contents of journals outside. Again this may be a better way of influencing soft power.

There are also lots of possibilities about publishing pieces on what it is like to work within your area of the Biological Sciences. This could be about your experience as an early career researcher, but may take on just about any stance that you feel is important in your area of Biological Sciences (e.g. language, covid, racism, colonialism, etc.).

5.4 Letters

These are generally very short pieces that you can write, often to high profile journals with letters pages. They can be used to raise the profile of all sorts of issues within your subject area or profession.

Letters are going to have to be polished and concise in order to get your point across in very few words.

5.5 Editorials

You are unlikely to be able to publish an editorial without first being an editor, but there may be a potential for you to become an editor, associate editor or junior editor in a number of society or publishers' journals. Once in position, the editorial is a powerful place to launch your opinion to subscribers.

There are such things as guest editorials for special issues and special issues are particularly useful if you are an early career researcher. If you want to edit a special issue of a journal in your area then approach the editor well in advance of when you want to do it (possibly more than a year in advance). It's often good to have these things linked to an event like a symposium that you are organising.

Once all the contents of the special issue are in, you can put an editorial together to explain what the idea was of the symposium and co-author it along with your other symposium organisers. Special issues of symposia often get cited more than other articles just because it is a collection of similar papers altogether in one place.

6

What is Impact Factor, and why is it so important?

The Impact Factor of a journal relates to the number of times each publication from the journal gets cited in the two years preceding the date of the Impact Factor (IF) (Equation 6). Thus, if you are thinking of publishing in a journal that has an IF of 1 you might expect that in the two years following the publication of your article you may get one citation. But as this is an average for all publications appearing in this journal, it is not necessarily true for your paper. As discussed elsewhere you might be very good at publicising your work and have it extensively cited. One or two extensively cited papers might even change the Impact Factor of the journal if it doesn't have so many publications per year. If on the other hand you are thinking of publishing your article in a journal that has an IF of 5, you might expect that your article will be cited five times more than if you published in the first journal (IF = 1).

It's a relatively simple calculation as seen in Equation (6):

$$\frac{\text{The sum of all citations in journal X for year Y}}{(\text{No. pubs in journal X for year Y}-1) + (\text{No. pubs in journal X for year Y}-2)}$$

Because all citations for year Y are needed before the IF can be calculated for each journal, IF for the preceding two years is typically not released until June of Y+1.

Impact Factors are published by a number of different literature databases. For example, for the Impact Factor calculated by the Web of Science (www.webofknowledge.com), if your journal is not even listed in the Web of Science then they will not assign any Impact Factor. The Web of Science is continually policing the quality of its journals, and this means from time to time journals are excluded. This tends to happen at the lower end of the Impact Factor scale. But recently it happened to some very well-known journals and there was a big stink (see Pinto et al. 2021).

Note that there are potential conflicts of interest with publishing Impact Factors. For example, a publisher, Elsevier, owns Scopus (www.scopus.com) and can decide whether or not a publication can get an Impact Factor in that database. Similarly, the new scholarly database, Dimensions (www.dimensions.ai), is

DOI: 10.1201/9781003220886-6

owned by Holtzbrinck who also own Springer Nature. Databases that are used by many of our employers in their means of evaluating our effectiveness are owned by for-profit companies. This is certainly cause for concern. There is a group of people who are trying to replace Impact Factor with a group of other metrics, so perhaps by the time you read this chapter, Impact Factor will no longer be relevant.

6.1   From a simple score to a way of life

When IF was originally devised by Eugene Garfield in 1955, it wasn't supposed to govern the lives of academics, it was simply intended to be a way of deciding which journals to include in the Science Citation Index (Garfield, 1999). It then became useful for librarians to help them decide which journals to keep and which to ditch under ever constrained budgets (caused by publishers' ever increasing prices). But along the way, this very simple index is now considered by many people to be a measure of quality, prestige and even academic success (Garfield, 1999). Many people have highlighted how wrong these beliefs are, but the growing trouble is that not only have many academics been misled, but so have administrators responsible for hiring and promotions.

"Like nuclear energy, the Impact Factor has become a mixed blessing."

—Eugene Garfield (1999)

A paper by McKiernan et al. (2019) found that IF features in the guidelines of many university panels responsible for the fate of academics' jobs and therefore lives. Worryingly, many of these institutions don't actually talk about what IF measures. Instead they equate it with values and qualities that it certainly does not represent. Thus, you may find that your career is influenced by a simple metric that almost all who use it don't actually understand. The undue influence on lives of scientists that IF has led directly to the San Francisco Declaration on Research Assessment (known as DORA) to which many institutions and publishers have signed up. You should read this very simple declaration and find out whether your institution is a signatory. If they are, then remember to hold them to the DORA principles during any assessment that you undergo.

The Impact Factor now dominates many aspects of life for Early Career Researchers, where the pay-off for a high impact publication might make the difference between having a job or leaving science altogether. The pressure is so high that it leads to misconduct and fraud.

6.2 Five-year Impact Factor

Many journals report their 'Five-Year Impact Factor' in addition to the standard two year timeframe (as seen in Equation 6). This is because many disciplines, such as Biological Sciences, don't have maximum impact of articles within the first two years of publication as do subjects like medicine and physics. Papers with immediate impact can be equated with sensational breaking news stories that instantly grab headlines, making money for those news outlets. These 'hot papers' or 'fast breaking papers' (i.e. left skewed distribution) will inflate the IF of the journal, which, if sustained, will earn the publisher more money. Most papers in Biological Sciences have a 'slow burn' (i.e. low frequency and long tails), consistently gathering small numbers of citations over long periods of time. Papers that suddenly become popular after a long time with no or very few citations are termed 'sleeping beauties' (i.e. right skewed; Bornmann and Marx, 2012). The last in the group of four citation types includes those that have a constant, usually low, number of citations over time. Together, each of these four patterns can be described by three variables that provide the citation behaviour of all papers: fitness, immediacy and longevity (see Fortunato et al., 2018). Using fitness, immediacy and longevity of citations to papers within a field can help to normalise citation metrics between different areas of science.

Although the five-year Impact Factor might be much more appropriate, most people ignore this metric. While this metric might be more appropriate, because of the bad ways in which people have used Impact Factor, it is probably better to push back against this metric as you should against others.

6.3 What can you do if you publish a journal with high IF?

Very high ranking journals for Impact Factor are publications like *Cell, Nature,* and *Science.* This is because these publications are read by a great number of people, and so are widely cited. Articles that get published in them receive a lot of attention from the press and media. This results in the prestige that a hiring institution might be looking for. For academics who publish in these journals, their institutions may well receive lots of positive publicity. In some countries, notably China, there may be a cash incentive towards publishing in a journal with a high IF (Quan et al., 2017).

One frightening trend that we are seeing in Biological Sciences is that the higher the Impact Factor the more the journal will charge you to publish in it. At the time of writing (November 2020) *Nature* has just announced that they will charge USD 9500 to publish Open Access in their highest-ranked journal (see Part II). This is more money than it cost to publish in any other journal at this moment, and will be greater than the cost of many research projects, or even salaries of Early Career Researchers in some parts of the world. There is a move for publishers to be transparent about what they charge to process articles, but the practices of the highest IF journals appear immoral.

6.4 Why is IF so important?

Academics are measured by their productivity but also on the quality of their output. Because there are so many different academic disciplines, the bean counters who administer us need some way of ranking academics against each other. This is why they use the Impact Factor of the journals in which their academics publish in order to determine the quality of their output. Even though there are other metrics of the actual quality of an academic, most administrators continue to cling to IF and their beliefs of what it stands for.

Some countries reward their academics if they publish in high ranking journals. This can result in a salary bonus (Quan et al., 2017). It may also help with promotion, getting tenure or even just getting an interview for a job (Schimanski and Alperin 2018; McKiernan et al. 2019). If you're going to publish and you want a career in academia then you need to be aware of Impact Factors and what they mean to different stakeholders.

Many people will complain that their particular sub-discipline has a range of very low ranking journals with low Impact Factors. Others complain that journals with high Impact Factors tend to be edited by an old boys club that facilitates the members. In some cases like *Proceedings of the National Academy of Sciences* this is certainly true.

6.5 Editors try to increase IF

It's important to remember that editors care about Impact Factor (see Ioannidis and Thombs, 2019). There are several reasons for this. Firstly, the Impact Factor of the journal can be used (by the publisher or society) as a simple measure of how well the editor is doing. Secondly, the higher the Impact Factor of the journal, the number of submissions of manuscripts increases so that the editor can select ones they perceive to be of higher 'quality'. Being the editor of a journal with a low (or no) Impact Factor can result in receiving fewer, more mediocre, manuscripts. Editors can only choose their content from what is submitted. Poor manuscripts take up much more time than good ones: more rounds of review, more disagreements among reviewers and more time spent making editorial decisions. Thus, by increasing the IF of the journal that you edit, you are likely to increase both the number of submissions (allowing you to reject poorer ones) and retain better ones.

All this means that if editors believe that your paper will not garner the same or more citations in two years as the current Impact Factor of their journal, they may desk reject your submission. This is just one of the ways in which editors are known to manipulate Impact Factors for their journals. Established ways (Metze, 2010; Martin, 2016) of editors increasing Impact Factor for their journals include:

- Ask authors to cite publications from their journal published within the last two years.
- Ask reviewers to suggest publications from their journal published within the last two years to authors on which their review is conducted.
- Encourage the submission of papers from laboratories with high output and citation rates.
- Reject papers that are likely to have no citations. This effectively reduces the size of the denominator in the above equation.
- Publishing issues in January means they have a maximum period of the year to get cited. This is now being inflated to having issues published online well ahead of the January date, all the time gathering citations.
- Encourage review articles which themselves garner more citations.
- Editorials that cite every paper in the journal. This tactic is frequently used in special issues.

6.5.1 Negotiating your IF

As the number of citations from your published content is divided by the number of papers, one way of improving the IF of a journal is to reduce the number of papers that are counted towards the denominator in the calculation made by the citations database. It has been known for some time that those journals with the highest IF negotiate the removal of all of their editorial and news content from their denominators, making the number of publications much smaller and hence the IF larger (Adam, 2002; Garfield, 1999). On the other hand, if any of these news articles or commentaries get citations, these are included in the addition to the numerator. Thus our favourite high impact journals, *Nature* and *Science*, can publish very citable news at the front of their magazine, but negotiate with the commercially minded database owners about exactly which of their content counts towards their IF (Brembs et al., 2013). Later, we will see evidence of the financial leverage that these negotiations can reward these top tier journals (see Part IV).

6.6 Push back against IF

Just like any metric, Impact Factor is liable for abuse. You need to be aware of how IF is used and abused by many people in the academic community. You also need to be aware of what the rewards are for these individuals. Our problem with Impact Factor is not really the way in which it is manipulated by individuals to achieve their own ends. Instead, we should be worried about the way in which it leads the scientific community towards bad science and dishonesty. People who have benefited from using IF to measure their careers are likely to object if their institutions abandon it (e.g. Chawla, 2021), even though they are already signatories of DORA. Retaining IF benefits these senior academics, their closed practices and the publishing industry who use this metric (that they own and police themselves) to direct money from taxpayers earmarked for research into their own pockets (more on this in Part IV).

If you must calculate IF, one very simple way that you can push back against industry-calculated IF is to calculate IF scores for your own papers, and show how they relate to the IF of the journal that you publish in. In this way, you are simply comparing your actual citations in the years (2 or more as appropriate) after your paper is published with the mean for the journal. There is an even chance that you generally get more citations than the mean for the journal, and you can convincingly show that your citations are consistently higher than the journal IF. For this to be true, you might need to help your work get cited, and that's the subject of another chapter.

7

When should you be an author?

Who should be an author is being increasingly regulated because of widespread abuse, including 'honorary authors' or excluding 'ghost authors'. Back in the day, there were people that used to add their pets to the author line including their dog, cat, hamster or parrot (Penders & Shaw, 2020)! One US physicist was so frustrated in being constantly rejected, that he added a fictitious Italian collaborator, Prof. Stronzo Bestiale from Palermo, Sicily (Penders & Shaw, 2020). Not only does Prof. Bestiale not exist, but stronzo bestiale means 'massive turd' in Italian. Another German physicist Prof. Alois Kabelschacht has co-authored a number of papers, but does not exist and is actually the German for 'cable duct' - a label next to a door in the Max Planck Institute for Physics in Munich, and regularly used as a straw man in the institute (Penders & Shaw, 2020). No doubt fictitious authors abound, but these are likely to come to an end with an increase in regulation.

These days we have ORCID that attempts to register all authors, turning them into numbers (see Part III). One of the benefits with the ORCID system is that you can have your name the way you want to have it, even if it is not a western style surname (Goyes Vallejos, 2021). The need for all this regulation is because publications have turned into a kind of currency for academics. And when there is currency involved, abuse quickly results in human systems followed by the need for regulation. Hence, one of the results of going transparent is that we all become registered numbers (and our dogs won't get authorship any more). Perhaps this is just the loss of an age of innocence, at least on the part of our pets!

A lot of the literature on the subject of ghost and honorary authorships has come from the medical profession, perhaps as this profession is prone to ghost authorship via the pharmaceutical industry (Matheson, 2016), and honorary authorship from heads of large research groups (see Rennie and Flanagin, 1994).

DOI: 10.1201/9781003220886-7

7.1   Ghost authorship

Ghost authorship is when people, not included in the author line, have contributed substantially to the study (Matheson, 2016). Note that ghostwriting outside science is usually when someone who has the talent to write, writes the ideas of someone who doesn't for a fee, and in return the latter takes the author line. These are called 'paper mills' and they are discussed later in Part I.

There are many potential sources for ghost authors, including past students whose thesis work is taken by unscrupulous advisors, and published without their inclusion. More commonly, I believe, is that those who contribute substantially are not included as authors for political reasons (they have fallen out of favour with those who are the authors), or they are simply forgotten because they have moved away from the institution. Ghost authorship is a land of the disenfranchised. This is becoming increasingly prevalent in the world of contributions of data, which is also freely accessible. Some authors will take and use the data, only referencing the DOI for where they obtained it. Others will include the original people who created the data as authors because they value their continued insight and input. Where the situation becomes very messy is when some people are included and others are excluded. This is my experience where a paper simultaneously contains honorary authors and excludes ghost authors. A study by Wisler et al. (2011) found ghost authorship in medical publications at 7.9%, although I'd argue that their methods (contacting corresponding authors) mean that the real levels are likely much higher.

While the world of inclusion (i.e. honorary authorship, see below) has a warm and friendly glow about it (everyone appears to benefit), exclusion is characterised by lack of information, contact and reasoning. If you are excluded from a publication even when you have contributed, you will not be getting an email from the authors detailing their decision. You'll be lucky if they even send you a copy once it's published. Meanwhile, those who are included will remain in the loop.

7.1.1   Paper mills

The concept of a paper mill is rather different from ghost authors or even salami-slicing (Part IV). Paper mills involve third parties, often not included on the author line, producing material for publication from scratch: i.e. companies that specialise in producing content that will pass peer review for those who want to buy authorship. The world of paper mills is particularly shady and it is not clear what sums of money are exchanged for these types of goods. A number of years ago there was evidence that first authorship on publications was for sale (Hvistendahl, 2013). What we do know is that there are benefits to those who are put on the authorline, while those that produce the manuscripts generally rewrite text and pull protocols from manuscripts that are already published. Results are often images that have already been published and/or are manipulated to suit the content (see Part IV). Hence, paper mills are a systematic and deliberate manipulation of the publication process (see Teixeira da Silva, 2021a).

7.2   Honorary authorship

Honorary authorship happens when people who have not contributed meaning-fully to a study are included in the author line. If publications are the currency of science then you can see how being added to other people's publications increases your apparent productivity. While this might sound surprising to you, you should know that it does happen and might be more common than you think. Wisler et al. (2011) found that honorary authorship was as high as 17.6% in medical publications. It's worth noting that this may vary between disciplines as there are various traditions in some disciplines whereby the head of a large team may always be included as an author of a paper that emerges from the team, whether or not they were involved: the White Bull effect (Kwok, 2005). In Biological Sciences, teams tend to be quite small with a single or rarely multiple Principal Investigators (PIs). This means that your PI will likely be directly involved with your research and therefore also an author. Imagine a very large team with multiple PIs working under a head who insists that they are an author on every publication. This could add up to hundreds of publications in a year (e.g. Yuri T. Struchkov is currently credited with >1600 publications on Scopus), and such prolific authorship has been questioned (e.g. Rennie and Flanagin, 1994). However, there appear to be very different levels of what could be considered credible and what incredible (e.g. 25 papers a year: Wager et al., 2015), and I respond to this, and the general question of how prolific authors are becoming, later in Part IV.

In the Biological Sciences, the area of molecular phylogenetics has traditionally honoured those who collect tissue samples with authorship on the resulting phylogenies when published. This is not always equal and has also been used to politically honour or ghost. The reason given for honouring contributors in this way is that the studies could not have been done without the tissues. On the other side, some people have long lists of publications based on tissue donations and very little else. What is needed is transparency.

7.3   A need for transparency – DORA

Given the problems with both ghost and honorary authorship, there is clearly a need for transparency about who the authors are and what they have actually contributed. This was recognised by the Declaration of Research Assessment (sfdora.org), which has a growing number of signatories as well as some solid ideas on the way forward in assessment of research and researchers. In particular, DORA is against the use of Impact Factors (see below) and other journal based metrics, and instead assesses the research on its own merits. DORA also encourages everyone to embrace the opportunities offered by online publication, including colour figures and unencumbered word lengths. DORA encourages specific information to be published about individual author contributions. In short, DORA stands for transparency and it would be worth you looking at their statement and finding out whether your institution is a signatory.

There are no universal rules about what or how much you should contribute in order to become an author of a scientific paper. However, some journals are independently initiating their own standards, and these might become more mainstream. Thus, it is worth discussing the criteria for being an author with your team preferably in a lab meeting so that everyone knows where they stand.

7.4   Who should be an author?

There is an increasing number of journals that now give clear instructions on who qualifies as author on a paper, and these have been formalised by the International Committee of Medical Journal Editors (ICMJE), and this area has been rapidly evolving (Baskin and Gross, 2011). Although these approaches are clearly made to prevent honorary authorships, it is hard to see how they help include ghosted authors or exclude the White Bull (Kwok, 2005). Scientists are notorious in their abilities to make *post hoc* rationalisations. As an early career researcher, I'd suggest that you use questions around authorship as a way to formulate how participating researchers fit into the study. By openly attributing roles to a checklist, everyone buys into what is expected of them. Any additions to this author line-up should be openly discussed amongst all authors, and attributed to the checklist, as the project proceeds.

7.4.1 Rescognito, ORCID and the CRediT Contributor Checklist

A new initiative under the name Rescognito (rescognito.com) has teamed up with ORCID to formally list the ways in which researchers are recognised per publication. Rescognito maintains the Data Availability Checklist, Contributor CRediT Checklist and Funder Information Checklist.

The CRediT Contributor Checklist (credit.niso.org) contains 14 fields:

Conceptualisation; Data curation; Formal Analysis; Funding acquisition; Investigation; Methodology; Project administration; Resources; Software; Supervision; Validation; Visualisation; Writing – original draft; Writing – review and editing.

Visit their website to learn more about these fields. This area has new initiatives and registries opening up. We will see how many journals adopt these and what becomes of existing initiatives in the future.

7.4.2 If you suspect irregularities in authorship

The Committee on Publication Ethics (publicationethics.org) (COPE) has published a useful flowchart to guide researchers on how to recognise potential authorship problems (COPE, 2018a). Or more specifically, how to recognise ghost, guest, or gift authorship in a submitted manuscript (Wager, 2006b).

8

Citations and metrics

Citations matter as they reflect the number of times your research was found to be useful. Although you can look at the citations of each paper, your publications will most likely be summarised into a citation metric to get an overview of how your work is used. Here I provide a guide to some of these metrics, how they are calculated and used. Throughout this book, I suggest that metrics should not be used to measure the performance of academics, and how the gamification of metrics has led to the detriment of the scientific project (see Chapman et al., 2019). However, you should be interested in the dissemination of your work, having it read as widely as possible, and ultimately cited when appropriate. Publishing your research in journals with higher Impact Factors will likely help you get your research read by a larger audience. But you can increase your own readership, and this chapter goes through some of ways in which you can disseminate your work and thereby increase the citations of your work wherever it is published.

8.1 What are your citation metrics?

A number of different databases compile metrics which you can access. In addition, they compile a bunch of extra performance metrics that you would have to pay to access, and in general these are available to a select number of recruitment staff at your institution. Here I will talk about Google Scholar, Scopus and the Web of Science (see Martin-Martin et al., 2018; Martín-Martín et al., 2021, on their differences). In summary, for Biological Sciences, the Web of Science (WoS) and Scopus are likely to give you very similar statistics. Scopus favours social-sciences a little more, so if your subject area does cross-over then you might see some extra citations there. Google Scholar is going to give you the highest metrics, but it doesn't mean that they are particularly false (although this is certainly not the best curated database). The joy of Google Scholar is that it is much more cosmopolitan on the journals and theses that it includes. So it actually gives you a better idea of who is using your research. It will also pick up grey literature and predatory publishers, so you should interpret the outputs with care.

DOI: 10.1201/9781003220886-8

Each of these databases offers you the opportunity of curating your own author profile that (in the case of Scopus and WoS) will link with your ORCID and (in the case of WoS) your Publons account. Your institution may want you to actively curate your profile to help them with assessing your institution's metrics. It is surprising how bad these are when left to the bots, especially if you have your name recorded in more than one way. I also think that it's worthwhile creating and curating a Google Scholar profile, and link it directly to your website. As an editor, this is one of the easiest ways of looking up an author or potential reviewer. For anyone that uses Google Scholar, your name will then be underlined, and other users can quickly find your other published works. Google Scholar also indexes preprints, which may be a boon to you as an Early Career Researcher.

Because all of these indices are cumulative, you can expect that anyone who started their career before you will have higher numbers. It is also worth being aware that some fields get higher citations because there are more people working in them, and therefore more articles are being published.

8.1.1 Total citations

Your total number of citations is simply the total number of times that anyone has cited one of your works within the respective database. Note that, the cited article itself doesn't have to appear in the database in order to be counted in total cites, but (clearly) the article that cites it must. For this reason, you are likely to have a different number of total citations in different databases.

8.1.2 H-index

Very simply, the H-index is the ranked count of the number of your publications that have received at least the same number of citations (Hirsch, 2005). The easiest way to calculate your H-index is to have a list of all your papers and their citations in a list, ranked from the highest to lowest cited (see Table 8.1). Counting down from the highest cited paper, you stop when the number of citations reaches the same as the numbered citation in the list. For example, your H-index will be 5 if you have authored 5 or more publications with 5 of them having received 5 citations or more. If 6 have received 5 citations, you'll still only have an H-index of 5, because for the H-index to grow to 6, the top 6 articles will need to be cited 6 times or more.

TABLE 8.1: A table of fictional papers ranked by their citations to show how H-index is calculated. In this table, the H-index is 5 as the 5th paper has 5 or more citations, and no other lower ranked paper has been cited >5 times. Note that the H-index is not 6 even though the 5th paper has 6 citations. Once the paper currently ranked 6 receives one more citation, the H-index of this author will rise to 6.

Rank	Title	Cited By	Year
1	A review of most important findings	48	2017
2	The first paper I presented at a conference	19	2017
3	Another significant finding	8	2018
4	First Open Access paper with snappy title	8	2020
5	**This paper spent a long time online first**	**6**	**2019**
6	Another review receiving some attention	5	2020
7	A paper that shows important findings	2	2020
8	Obscure note that I managed to self-cite	1	2018
9	The only citation is my own	1	2019
10	Hot off the press	0	2021
—	**Total Citations**	**98**	—

Your H-index will grow very quickly as you publish articles from your thesis, but the growth slows as the H-index grows as it requires more citations of particular papers (of your top cited papers). Growing an H-index is therefore very difficult, and it's probably one of the hardest of these metrics to manipulate. Because the H-index is cumulative, people with very large H-indices (>100) are usually very senior academics with very good networks, and low R numbers (see below).

Note that while the H-index is usually calculated for individuals, groups of people can also have an H-index, such as a department, a school, faculty or even university. Indeed, you can calculate an H-index for any set of articles using the citations that they receive.

8.1.2.1 Normalisaing the H-index and other citation metrics

The H-index (and other indices) are sometimes normalised for field of study (fixed – dynamic; broad – narrow), types of citing documents and year of publication (see Ioannidis et al., 2016). You can expect to see some of these field normalisations, for example by Dimensions (see Figure 8.1) who provide you with, total citations (as the name implies), recent citations (citations within the last 2 years), field citation ratio (comparing the article to ones of a similar age in in a similar field) and the relative citation ratio (relative to 1.0, this gives you an idea of how well cited the article is compared to others in its area of research). As an Early Career Researcher, you may feel that your H-index is not particularly impressive (Table 8.1), in which case, you may want to consider some of these normalised metrics if they show your articles in a more favourable light.

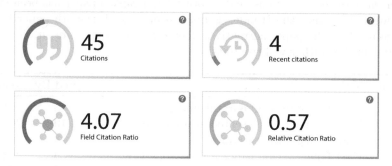

FIGURE 8.1: Normalising citation metrics. Some databases will provide you with normalised values for citations, like the one shown here by Dimensions for a paper cited 45 times, and 8% of these citations are from the past two years (normalised for time since published). The Field Citation Ratio (FCR) of this paper is 4.07 times more citations, when compared to other papers in the field. The Relative Citation Ratio (RCR) compares this paper to other NIH-funded publications in the same area of research and year, where they will be the same as the mean (at 1.0), more or (in this case) less at 0.57.

8.1.3   G-index

The G-index is similar to the H-index, but places more emphasis on the actual number of citations in your top cited articles (Egghe, 2006). To calculate this, you will need to organise your publications by the number of times that they have been cited. For ease of explanation, start with your H-index, and add up citations to all of the preceding articles (1st, 2nd, 3rd, 4th and 5th). For example, in order for your G-index to be 5, all citations up to 5 will need to be more than or equal to 25 (5^2). For your G-index to increase to 6, the sum of all citations to your first 6 papers will need to be equal or greater than 36 (6^2). Our fictional researcher in Table 8.1 has a G-index of 9 as citations to the first 9 articles add up to 98 which is greater than 81 (i.e. $>9^2$).

Because the G-index uses all citations in your top cited articles, not simply the minimum used to obtain the H-index, your G-index should be equal or higher than your H-index. This is because of the phenomenon that articles that get cited more, continue by getting increasing numbers of citations (known as the Matthew Effect, see below). Therefore, you may favour using the G-index if your top papers are particularly well cited.

8.1.4 R-index

Your R-index is a measure of your active network (Ioannidis, 2008). It is rather like the H-index in that it records the count of the number of people that you've collaborated with on a number of papers. But these need to be the same people. This is then divided by your total number of papers. For example, if your thesis produced 5 papers with the same 5 authors and this is your total number of papers, your R-index will be 1. However, if two of the papers lacked one of the people, your R-index will drop to 1.66. If you don't work with those 5 other people again, then your R-index will grow continuously until you have another productive network. See the section on networks for a fuller explanation of the R-index and the importance of networks.

8.1.5 a-index

The a-index is calculated from the total number of citations divided by H^2 (Sidiropoulos et al., 2007). In the example given in Table 8.1, Total citations is: 98. H^2 is 25 (5^2), and so the a-index is $98/25 = 3.92$. This index gives a measure of how top-heavy someone's citations are. The a-index gets larger as the highest ranked papers receive a disproportionate amount of citations. This is known as the Matthew Effect (see below), and this is a general feature of a lot of researchers' citation ranks.

8.1.6 i10-index

Your i10 index represents the number of articles that you have written which have been cited 10 times or more in that database. The i10 is often expressed over a time frame (e.g. the last 5 years) which may well exclude papers that you write that have an immediate but not a lasting impact. Moreover, looking at an index calculated over the last 5 years will let you know how active citations for older papers are. Given that most indices are cumulative, older researchers almost always look better. But a time constrained index may provide additional insight into their relative productivity.

8.1.7 Other metrics

There are more metrics for authors behind paywalls, but there are also metrics on social media sites such as ResearchGate's 'RG score'. The way that ResearchGate calculates its RG score is rather opaque and is not simply done on publication metrics, but on the way that you interact with your ResearchGate community. Similarly, many publishers will grant you metrics that will be boosted by the number of times that you publish with them. Many researchers eschew scores, such as the RG score, as there is no transparency in how this is calculated.

There are also Altmetrics handed out as a means of showing the alternative impact for articles that you've written. These are explained in Part III.

8.2   How to increase your citations

Increasing your total number of citations is likely to impact positively on all of your metrics, but this is not necessarily true, and hence why you may be assessed on more than one metric. In the following subsections, I go through some of the well-known ways in which you can increase the readership of your paper, and with this the likelihood that someone will cite it.

8.2.1   Media release

Some journals will want you to write a media release that they may use to promote your paper. You can also proactively write a press release and send it to the media office at your institution. Writing a release for the media is very different from scientific writing, and you can find a guide in Part III.

8.2.2   Social media

Social media is another way of getting your article to the attention of more people. Twitter has been adopted by many scientists and tweeting out an article that gets retweeted by the right people (i.e. social media hubs – with lots of followers) can get you tens or even hundreds of thousands of views. This is likely to be far in excess of anything your article will get by passively sitting on the journal website.

At this point it is worth telling the tale of Neil Hall, who in 2014 wrote a slightly mischievous short article proposing a new citation metric which he called the **K-index** to reflect the number of followers on Twitter divided by the total number of citations of the same researcher (Hall, 2014). In the article, he found (with a non-random selection of 40 researchers on Twitter) that there was indeed a correlation between well-cited individuals and the number of their Twitter followers. He then postulated that some people with large numbers of Twitter followers (high celebrity) were not authoritative as they did not have lots of citations (a measure of scientific value):

> "... a high K-index is a warning to the community that researcher X may have built their public profile on shaky foundations,..."
>
> — Neil Hall (2014)

A social media backlash followed swiftly. Within days of the online publication, the Tweets started rolling in, with a great many people very upset with what they saw as an insult to younger researchers who had a good social media following on Twitter (Woolston, 2014). The social media eruption over this article gave it an Altmetric score of 2489, ranked 1st among the articles published at that time in that journal, and 9th in all journals. Although Hall had written the article in a light hearted way (poking fun at metrics and social media), the backlash was massive (although some did appreciate the joke).

There are several lessons here: First, what seems like a joke to you (including those immediately around you) may be offensive to others, especially those from other cultures. Second, items in social media can go badly wrong, and be taken in ways that you had never imagined. Third, social media goes well beyond academia – as is the intention with the dissemination, and that this may also have repercussions.

The bottom line is that social media can be an excellent way to reach a very wide audience, but that you must use it responsibly, or risk that it might do you and your reputation considerable damage.

8.2.2.1 Academic social media sites

Sites such as ResearchGate and Academia.edu will play a role in increasing citations to your work, especially if you have a large following. Rather like sharing on traditional social media sites, the more people who are exposed to your work, the more likely they are to read and cite it. In the case of academic social media sites, the audience is more niche and so more likely to find your work of interest.

8.2.3 Popular articles

Writing popular articles is a good way to ensure that your paper gets some media attention. There are outlets like The Conversation (theconversation.com) that specialise in publishing popular articles written by academics. But you

might also find that academic societies that you belong to have newsletters
that you can contribute a popular article to about your paper. As long as the
circulation of these newsletters is big, it should enhance the numbers of people
that eventually read about your work.

8.2.4   Self-citations

Self citation is when you cite a paper that you or one of your co-authors have
written or co-authored. This is probably one of the oldest and most widely
practised ways of increasing citations to your articles. It is generally frowned
upon to have gratuitous self-citations, but the situation may be complex and
biased (see Flatt et al., 2017).

It is also true that you are more than likely to cite your own work because you
have probably published in the same area previously. By the end of a typical
PhD, for example, you will already be citing publications that you produced at
the beginning. Self-citations are also known to facilitate the 'Matthew effect',
whereby because you increase your level of citations of a particular paper,
others will also cite it (Fowler and Aksnes, 2007; Flatt et al., 2017). There is
evidence to suggest that the proportion of self-citations will change in different
disciplines, and that they will increase with increasing numbers of collaborative
co-authors (Davarpanah and Amel, 2009). Self-citations are also known to
increase with increasing career length (Mishra et al., 2018), presumably with
the growth of one's own publication base in relevant areas. Because of this
effect, self-citation can be regarded as a measure of highly productive authors
(Mishra et al., 2018).

There has even been a call for another metric, the **s-index** which is the
equivalent of the h-index but for self-citations (Flatt et al., 2017): 'the total
number of s papers that an author has published that have at least the same
amount of s self-citations'.

How do you make sure that self-citations citations are not gratuitous? Simply
by only citing a paper when you need to. Note that many citation indices
will provide your citation scores both with and without self-citations. As a
rule of thumb, metrics suggest reasonable levels self-citations in the Biological
Sciences are ~30% (Aksnes, 2003). In short, there is nothing wrong with citing
yourself, but you should only do so when you need to.

8.2.5   Citing papers submitted and in press

If you, or others, have papers that are 'in press', then you can cite these in a
manuscript submitted to a journal for peer review. However, 'in press' does
mean that they have been formally accepted by an editor at a journal. These

days, the concept of 'in press' is not quite the same as it was. It used to take months before an accepted paper would appear in a journal issue. These days it is likely that you'll have an online version very quickly after acceptance. Hence, by the time you submit a manuscript with citations to papers that are 'in press', by the next round of revisions or acceptance, they should be fully available. If papers are not available by the time you send back your proofs, then you may well be asked to remove these citations. My impression is that many authors claim that a paper is 'in press' when the reality is that it's simply been submitted and that they are hoping it will be 'in press'.

You should not add citations to manuscripts that have simply been submitted to other journals. If you really need to, then submiting and citing as a preprint is really your only option. Some editors will not accept citations of preprints. An exception to this might be when papers are submitted together to the same journal at the same time. If this is the case, then you can point this out to the editor in your cover letter.

If the contents of another manuscript are pivotal for understanding the submitted version, then you should make sure that there is a copy of the 'in press' or 'submitted' manuscript available for the reviewers. The easiest way of doing this will be as a preprint. If this is not possible, then you may need to upload the manuscript as an additional file – but you should seek guidance from the journal editor.

8.2.6 Presenting the results of your paper at a conference

Probably the most traditional way of generating a bigger audience for your work is to talk about it (or present it as a poster) at a conference with an audience that is likely to appreciate your work. Everyone else at the conference will likely also be wanting you to know their work, so you'll need to target your audience carefully (possibly in a symposium), and make sure that the audience can access your work (e.g. through a QR code in your slide or on the poster). Making your talk memorable will likely have people recall your work, and cite it if they are undertaking a similar or relevant study.

8.2.7 Organising symposia and having special issues

Having your research published in a special issue is a great way of getting citations. This is because special issues have research on a theme and so many people will be drawn to the issue and are then more likely to see your work. This includes other people who participate in the special issue and are *de facto* already interested in this line of research. This increased visibility of your research is, in my opinion, a good reason for joining a special issue if you have the chance.

Special issues are often edited by people who have an interest in pulling together this kind of research. They may encourage other authors in the special issue to cross cite articles, and may write an editorial that includes citations to yours and other papers. Of course, the best position to be in is when you are one of the organising members. Your name will be associated with the special issue as well as your contribution. This means that when the special issue is published, each of the papers in it will already have citations leading to a positive Matthew Effect from day one of publication.

Probably the easiest way of pulling together a special issue is to organise a symposium at a conference and ask those participating to contribute to the special issue. If this is done long enough in advance and you are good at organising then it can work very well. Talk to your mentor about the possibility of their help in organising a symposium.

8.2.8 Traditional media

To get your work cited you need to get people reading it. As scientists read the traditional media, it can be a way of bringing your work to their attention, and result in additional citations. There are other benefits of having your work highlighted by the traditional media. You should always make sure that you get a plug in for your institution and any prominent funders. There are now additional metrics (e.g. Altmetrics) that track traditional and social media and in the future you might be able to use these altmetrics to your advantage in getting a job, a promotion or tenure.

8.2.9 Not-so-legitimate ways of increasing citations

Apart from the legitimate ways of increasing citations and visibility of your work that I've listed above, there are other illegitimate ways that I have heard about. I have heard of certain laboratories that have *quid pro quo* arrangements where they agree to cite each other's publications (see Ritchie, 2020).

Another way of increasing citations might be to have a co-author who is very well-known. Certainly having a co-author who is very well-known is likely to increase your citations but only if they actually do something to contribute to the work. See the section on honorary authorship.

Gratuitous self-citations. As mentioned above, you should really only cite your own work when necessary, and not more than this.

Journals have also been known to manipulate citations in order to increase their Impact Factors and therefore their perceived level of quality. A group of physics journals from Romania were found to have clearly manipulated self-citations to increase their own Impact Factors (see Heneberg, 2016). There can also be a level of coercive pressure from journal editors to cite papers from their journals published within the two year citation window (Chorus and Waltman, 2016). Such practices are now systematically analysed by the larger literature databases, and clear levels of Impact Factor manipulation result in delisting of the journal from the database.

8.3 Well-cited articles are likely to be cited more

Articles that already have a lot of citations are more likely to pick up extra citations than the ones that have very few. This phenomenon, sometimes referred to as the Matthew Effect (see Teixeira da Silva, 2021b; Merton, 1968), is exaggerated by search engines like Google Scholar that order the results of searches by the number of times an article is cited. Like people looking for a website, academics looking for a paper are more likely to choose one on the first page of Google Scholar than to keep searching through Google Scholar until they find your study. In effect, this means that those that already have large research groups and that can generate initial citations, will get more citations and increase their own standing. Or, in other words, those that are already in a commanding position will automatically generate more (Casadevall and Fang, 2012) – the winner takes it all.

As you read through papers in your specialist area you will notice that there are some papers that seem to get cited over and over again as standard examples of a particular phenomenon. These are often some of the first examples published and have also been published in higher ranking journals. If you are the 20th person to have shown a particular phenomenon then it is unlikely that your paper is going to end up being cited the most.

There have been investigations into what makes certain papers more likely to be cited further. One of the factors that appears to be significant is the 'small-study effect' – low precision studies that produce large effect sizes, either spuriously (i.e. a Type I error: Forstmeier et al., 2017) or genuinely (Fanelli et al., 2017).

9

Growing your network

During your PhD you will have had an advisor who would have been central to many of the decisions that you made. Don't give up on that relationship, it is something that you have at the heart of your network. Therefore it is worth maintaining the best professional relationship possible, as this is someone who you will need to go back to (probably lots of times) for references and other professional help. In short, always keep your advisor sweet. The same could be said about your thesis committee members, if you had one.

Having said this, as an early career researcher, you are now advisor-less, yet it is likely that you will still need advice from someone more experienced. Hopefully, there will always be your advisor, but the chance is that you may well have changed institutions, and so they may not be so close or easy to contact. This is a good reason for expanding your network by looking for a mentor to your role as an early career researcher. Increasing numbers of institutions are now recognising that early career researchers need mentors to advise them about how to move forward within their academic field. Moreover, mentors can help promote equality and inclusively (Davies et al., 2021).

9.1 What to look for in a mentor

The first thing to look for in a mentor is someone that you feel you are able to talk to easily. As you will see, there are a wide range of topics to discuss in terms of building your career, and you will need to find someone that you feel you can talk to about nearly everything safely and without fear that it might be used against you. The mentor should feel happy to talk and spend time with you. They should be someone that is genuine in their desire to help you and your career. You won't have a fruitful relationship with someone that doesn't really like you, or doesn't want to spend time talking to you.

Next, your mentor should be someone who is already well established within an academic network that you want to (or already are) a member of. You will need to have common ground to talk about, and getting their advice on building your network will necessitate talking about how to manage others in the network.

The personal touch is nice to have, so if you can find a mentor who has an office in the same building, or on the same campus, then it's great to be able to meet up and chat. However, your mentor doesn't have to be in the same institution, or even in the same country. In these days of post-pandemic communication we are all a lot happier hooking up to meetings online.

If you still have choices, my suggestion would be to look for someone who you share non-academic interests with. For example, you may both enjoy playing squash together, hiking or scuba-diving. Meeting outside academia will make your mentor-mentee chats easier for both of you. Otherwise, try not to make your meetings with your mentor a burden on their work time. All academics are busy and core-working hours are hard to come by. Instead you could suggest taking your mentor out for a coffee or a sandwich during which you have your chat.

Note that a mentor doesn't have to be someone that is particularly senior, although they should be well connected. Having said this, they are likely to be at a more advanced career stage than you.

9.2   Questions to put to your mentor

Your mentor's time is valuable, so always have an agenda when you go to talk to them. Have ideas that you want to pitch and get feedback from. Have some way of making notes about what they say, especially if you meet over a beer. You don't want to have to go back and ask them again for the same advice. Be prepared to get the answer that they give. This seems an odd thing to say, but they may not always like your idea, and you should be prepared to listen to their advice whatever it is, not only when it agrees with your own ideas.

Typical things to discuss with your mentor are:

- Where to publish
- What meeting to attend
- How to extend your network
- Whether (or not) to write a reply or commentary on another groups' work
- Whether to respond to a call for grant applications
- Whether to apply for a job

You may also want to share some of the more exciting aspects of your work, your findings and how you interpret them. Try to keep away from moaning about other academics, the amount of administration you have, teaching burdens, etc. Make your discussions as positive as possible so that your mentor is more likely to want to maintain and grow the relationship.

9.3   The importance of networks in your academic career

There is clear evidence that researchers with good networks collaborate more, publish more and are better cited (Fortunato et al., 2018; Parish et al., 2018). Your mentor can be one way to increase your academic network. Perhaps more importantly, they can be a guide to help you through the network that you are involved with.

There is a good chance that you are already in a network where your advisor, and perhaps some members of your thesis committee, sit at the hub of an extended network that you have had partial exposure to during the course of your studies. If you haven't realised already, these networks are of profound importance in every step of your academic career. Evidence from studies on the science of science (SciSci) suggest that within networks there is a great importance for small teams to disrupt science (Fortunato et al., 2018). In order to find team members (and for them to find you), you need to have a network of people to draw from.

Benefits of a good network include:

- increased citations for your work
- better chances that your work will be edited or reviewed by a member or an associate of your network, resulting in a higher chance of publication or a grant application accepted
- increased potential to be nominated for an award
- increased potential to be invited to give talks at conferences
- invitation to apply for positions and jobs in the labs of partners at institutions in the network

If you are already in a network, you should be thinking of ways in which you can get more from your network now that you are an early career researcher. If, on the other hand, you are not in a good (sizeable and supportive) network, you should be thinking about how to join an existing network or how to form a network around yourself and your work.

In many cases, managing your network is about providing opportunities for yourself and others in your network. There are many ways in which you can do this, but you should be prepared to put in a lot of work from your own side.

Potential initiatives include:

- writing a grant application that involves others in your network
- leading a piece of written work that includes others in the network
  - a review
  - a commentary on another article (not from your network!)
  - a viewpoint or position article on an emerging topic
- organising a symposium aimed at a central or emerging question within your network
- organising a special issue of a journal (potentially as a result of the symposium)

Your chosen mentor is the best person to discuss how to make positive waves in your network. Remember that relationships have already been forged in networks and you should never try to destabilise these. Instead, you should aim to become another node of the network by growing your own usefulness as a positive force for new and interesting initiatives that others will want to join. Because you are new, don't expect to be included in every initiative. If you feel that you are being unnecessarily left out of other initiatives that you've heard about, ask your mentor whether or not it is appropriate for you to bring this up.

Always bridge and build relationships. As you should have become aware by now, there are many potential ways of becoming involved in combative elements of academic life. Your own sub-discipline will likely have groups of people that write commentaries about the work of other groups. Networks are powerful places to be, but they can also become destructive when another network opposes a position. I have seen this type of behaviour happen within and around my own limited subdisciplines. One group will publish a major finding in *Nature* or *Science* and a week or two later, the other group will publish a commentary pointing out what are (to them) flaws in the first group's publication. I always have a sneaking admiration for those individuals that appear to swim between these groups, always maintaining good relationships with both sides. Theirs is really an interesting, but perhaps precarious, position.

If you feel that you don't have any network, then I think that you should reassess your position. You likely do have people that you talk to and interact with that are already part of a network, but your question is how to increase the size, and potential scope, of your network. In the same way that everyone will have their own path through their career, the best way to grow your network will be unique to you.

9.3.1   Calculating the size of your network

A simple metric for your network is the total number of co-authors that you have from all of your publications. Clearly, as you increase the number of people that you work and (hopefully) publish with, you will have a bigger, better functioning network. However, scientometricians have their own ways of interpreting and mapping networks (see Figure 9.1).

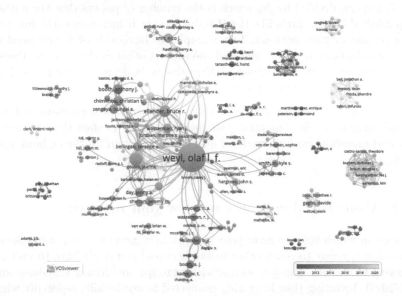

FIGURE 9.1: An author network for the Web of Science search for 'Invasive fish' AND 'South Africa'. In this author network you will see my friend and colleague, the late Prof. Olaf Weyl, who is at the centre of a large group of people who worked on invasive fish in South Africa. Olaf's wasn't the only research group, but certainly the most influential and joined up. Olaf's collaborations were extensive, spanning continents and generations of researchers. Drawn with VOSviewer (van Eck and Waltman, 2010).

If you aren't sure about who's in what networks within your own researcher area, you can use appropriate keywords to download literature within the area that you work, and plot (using VOSviewer: van Eck and Waltman, 2010) a similar author and co-author network. I'd suggest using enough keywords to call ~1000 articles (including their citations) that include your research area (all or the majority of your papers should be included). Using a *map based on bibliographic data*, read the bibliometric files and analyse using co-authorship to describe the linkages between authors. This can be very revealing (see Figure 9.1), and while you should already be well aware of the big names in your area, some of the people that span areas and sub-subdisciplines might well be worth seeking out. When looking into their publications, ask yourself how they managed to span between networks (conducting a postdoc in each lab is one such way). More than this, you can use collaborations to combine networks of other Early Career Researchers in your subject area.

Another method for determining the size of your network, or those of potential collaborators around you, is to calculate your R value (Ioannidis, 2008). **R** is made up of two figures, I_1 which is the number of authors that appear in at least I_1 papers, divided by N_p which is the number of papers that the author has published. I_1 is a little like the H-index in that it increases each time you add a person in your network. For example, to have a I_1 of 4, you need at least 4 publications in which you and the same 4 other authors occur. Parish et al. (2018) show that as I_1 grows, so the value of **R** decreases and researchers become most productive as **R** approaches 1.

Once you start to calculate your own value of **R**, you will appreciate that not only are large networks important, but that it is useful to start these networks early and maintain working with an every increasing group throughout your career.

9.3.2   Using social networks to grow your network

The ways in which you can grow your network have never been so great. Social networking is a way to reach other researchers and you don't have to wait for a meeting to do this. The #academictwitter groups are already very large and established. Investing time in getting connected is worthwhile, especially when you can meet up in person through conferences and symposia. I don't want to make out that Twitter, and (no doubt) other social networking is easy, but it is a good way of hooking up with a whole lot of other people without having to leave your desk. You can pitch ideas, and get collaborations moving in your area. Once you have it working for you, it is very empowering; remaining aware that it can go wrong. If social networking is your thing, then I'd suggest trying to find yourself a 'social networking mentor' – someone who already has a good following and can guide you through the various nuances of (often unspoken) rules that happen on these platforms.

9.4   Creating your own website

Whether or not you have your own lab as an Early Career Researcher you would be doing yourself a favour by creating your own website. Having a website is a way of creating your own brand and making you distinct from whatever institution or group you are a member of.

Websites don't have to be fancy. There are plenty of ways in which to make good-looking websites using templates (Weebly, Wix, etc.). You can make these unique to you simply by using your own photographs. If you're not a photographer then consider using some of the images from your work, or ask a colleague whether you can use some of theirs. Remember to place the most important keywords for your area in the website metadata so that it will pop up in any general web searches. There's a lot of information out there on how to build a successful website that people can find, so I won't go into this here.

What to include on your website

- Make sure that you have your professional contact details, including your institutional email address. This will help any editors for other colleagues that are trying to contact you. Avoid having a form as the only way of making contact with you.
- Write some general blurb about yourself and your work including all relevant keywords for your subject area.
- Have a list of your publications, conference presentations, popular articles, patents and any other outputs that are relevant to your professional profile.
- Provide a summary of your professional research experience listing where you did your degrees and any post-doctoral work.
- Make sure that your website works on lots of different platforms. Preferably it will work on mobile devices as well as desktops and laptops.
- Link to your various academic profiles: Publons, ORCID, Scopus, Research-Gate, Academia.edu, GitHub, etc.
- Provide a link back to your institutional website and your current lab, as this will help legitimise your independent website standing. People want to see that you are who you claim to be.

Optional items

- You could write a blog
- You could have short articles about some of your publications
- Downloadable version of your CV
- Future plans for projects
- Collaborator page – with links to collaborators in your network
- Data from projects (e.g. images, sounds, videos, R code, etc.)

Things to avoid

- Be careful about mixing personal and professional profiles
- Don't provide links to any personal social media accounts, only professional ones
- Don't allow your site to be too static (static sites rank lower in search results)

10

Preprints

10.1 What are preprints?

So far in this book, I have explained about the process of peer review and how important it is, and later I explain why it's the silver (and not gold) standard in science. Preprints came to us from the world of physics. An academic world that is moving so quickly that many inside it don't want to wait for peer review before making their work public. They date back to 1991, and were the brainchild of Paul Ginsparg with his preprint server, *arXiv*. Today, *arXiv* hosts nearly 2 million articles in 8 subject areas: Physics, Mathematics, Computer Science, Quantitative Biology, Quantitative Finance, Statistics, Electrical Engineering and Systems Science and Economics.

In addition to making your work open access, it allows anyone to read and review it. This is unlike the traditional publishing model where editors invite selected reviewers. Many consider preprints as a kind of open peer-review system.

> "The life science community needs to return to a culture of evaluating scientific merit from reading manuscripts, rather than basing judgment on where papers are published."
>
> –Ron Vale (2015)

In Biological Sciences the most prominent preprint server is called *bioRxiv* (www.biorxiv.org).

DOI: 10.1201/9781003220886-10

10.2 Who posts preprints on *bioRxiv*?

In an analysis by Abdill and Blekhman (2019) back in 2018, there were 37,648 preprints uploaded to *bioRxiv*. But in the world of preprints, this information is quite dated as back then there were only ~2,000 uploads each month. Luckily, these same authors regularly scrape data regarding submissions to *bioRxiv* and I reproduce these data below. It is interesting to look at the concern back in 2015 that preprint servers like *bioRxiv* might not catch on in the Biological Sciences (Vale, 2015), and it is still true to say that the number of preprints in the life sciences is still dwarfed by the annual number of publications, whereas physics has seen the opposite trend.

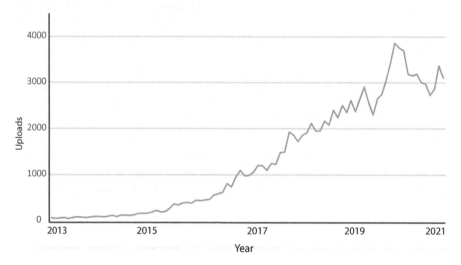

FIGURE 10.1: The growth of *bioRxiv* submissions in time. Note how the rate of submission rocketed at the beginning of the pandemic lockdown, and has remained high ever since.

What you see is a doubling of *bioRxiv* submissions dating back to May 2020 (Figure 10.1), a few months after the start of the global COVID-19 pandemic. (Go to the RXivist website (rxivist.org/stats) to see the incredible spike in medRxiv (www.medrxiv.org) data at the same point in time.) Many scientists had spent a few months working from home. Some had been productive and many decided to move this productivity for the first time onto *bioRxiv*.

In answer to the question above, **just about everyone now posts preprints on *bioRxiv*.** Those that don't likely use other preprint servers, or are not moving with the times.

The preprint revolution has not gone unnoticed by the tech giants. Back in 2017 the Chan Zuckerberg Initiative made an undisclosed donation to *bioRxiv*. The advisory board also has the architect for Google Scholar, Anurag Acharya.

10.3 Why might you want to post a preprint?

One of the advantages of posting a preprint is that it gets a DOI (digital object identifier www.doi.org). You can then use this DOI to refer to your work even though it is not published in a peer review journal.

For example, imagine that you've just finished your thesis and only one of your chapters is published. How can you show to prospective employers how good your work is? Or if you are applying for money how can you refer to your work even though it's not published? A preprint is a simple solution to this problem.

Other benefits include having a wider scope of peer reviewers. If you know that in your subject area there are many people who may want to comment on your work constructively, then this would be an opportunity to give them access. Importantly, because a preprint has a DOI, your work is not vulnerable to theft. It also allows you to stake your claim on the work that you've already done even though there may be a lag time between this and it coming out in a journal with full peer review.

If you do want feedback on a manuscript that you have posted as a preprint then you will need to tell people about it. A good example of this would be after providing a talk, or a poster, at a conference you might show a QR code where people can read your manuscript as a preprint. You can also publicise it to your community on social networks like Twitter.

If you get lots of feedback on your manuscript then you should expect to incorporate it. So be careful what you wish for, because you could be opening yourself up for a lot of comments.

Posting a preprint on *bioRxiv* is also a shortcut to submission to a growing number of traditional journals. Manuscripts and Supplementary Information can be transmitted directly from the preprint server to many journals without the need to upload the files and metadata a second time.

10.4   Upload newer versions

If you, or others, spot errors in your preprint, or you find new literature to
cite, you can update your manuscript with a new version. Indeed you should
do this for as long as your preprint remains active. Once published, make sure
that there is a pointer from your preprint to the published version.

10.5   Will you have to post a preprint?

This field is moving quickly. In December 2020, at least one journal (*eLife*
'publish then review') announced that they won't accept a submission until a
preprint has been registered. Thus all reviews are made on preprints. Other
journals, like *PLoS*, are announcing in house preprint servers. You should
expect this area to rapidly change in the coming years, so no matter when you
are reading this, you are more likely than ever to need to submit a preprint.

At the time of writing, there are still some journals that make it a condition of
submission that there is no preprint. Make sure you check within your target
journal list.

If you choose to publish in an overlay journal, then you'll have to deposit your
submission onto a preprint server.

10.6   Could these comments pages really replace peer
review?

Peer review is often regarded as a gold standard in scientific publishing (although a silver standard would be more realistic), and there's certainly a lot
to that. It ensures that published material has been read and its contents
assessed independently. But peer review is fallible, because scientists are all
humans. These problems are discussed at length in Part IV.

In 2003, Stefano Mizzaro proposed changing peer review to the format that
we now see in preprint journals (Mizzaro, 2003). Let every reader become a
reviewer. Another take on this same theme is provided by Heesen and Bright
(2020) who argue for a more subtle change in the date of publication (prior

to peer review as seen in preprints) instead of after peer review. Here their emphasis is on removing the wasted time spent reviewing and then rejecting manuscripts that will never be published. Their discourse is very persuasive, yet given that both models currently exist, we need more ideas on how we could drive a preprint model forward. More ideas do exist, and I encourage you to explore those proposed in a special issue edited by Kriegeskorte et al. (2012).

In the preprint model, several peer review problems might be overcome as no-one chooses the reviewers. Instead they choose themselves, and are motivated to do the work. Their competence to cover all aspects of the manuscript is not assured, but one assumes that independently motivated reviewers will only comment on parts that they are able to assess.

All of this is very good, but will people actually read and comment? A quick look at the sites will tell you a lot about the level of reviewing that is currently going on in biosciences preprints. Looking at the top 10 articles on *bioRxiv* (zoology section in November 2020) confirmed my suspicions. Plenty of tweets about the articles, but none of them had any comments, let alone reviews. Indeed, a further trawl through *PeerJ Preprints*, also found no comments.

When reviewers aren't chosen, there's potential for manipulation. This could promote a culture for comments to preprints for well-known labs, and (conceivably) a certain amount of trolling for labs with ongoing disputes or rivalries. This would make preprint peer review a sort of trial by popularity. But I don't see a situation where potential reviewers will take time-out once a week (for example) and hunt for manuscripts that have received no comments. It seems far more likely that the authors will have reciprocal agreements with other groups to review each other's manuscripts. This nepotistic tendency then puts us back into the area of problems in peer review that we've been working hard to overcome now for sometime.

10.7 Preprints are here to stay

It is clear that preprints are with us to stay. The year of the COVID-19 pandemic (2020) saw an explosion of preprint papers on the topic, but also saw the misunderstanding of what these articles mean by the press and general public alike. Rapid sharing of results via preprint servers has already been put in place following the outbreak of Zika virus in South America (back in 2015-16), but the global nature of the COVID-19 public health crisis saw much larger numbers of preprints being placed online.

But the value of preprints will always be limited for as long as there is no peer review. Moreover, comments won't suffice for peer review as there is no editorial oversight. As you'll read elsewhere, the role of the editor is pivotal in publishing.

10.8   When should evaluation end?

One point raised many times in the special issue edited by Kriegeskorte et al. (2012) is that evaluation should be open-ended: **ongoing evaluation**. There was a consensus to see reviewers continue to question the contents of papers long after publication. But these authors don't appear to have a realistic perspective on the time taken by authors to rebut their work. Imagine the effort that you currently put into a rebuttal letter. Now consider that your first rebuttal might come after a few months, and then you need to compose another after a few years. Perhaps you are the only author still working (especially if it is the work of your students). Perhaps all of your co-authors are dead! Suddenly you are called upon to defend your work, potentially decades after completion. Can you do it? Would you want to do it? What would be the consequences of not doing it? Would people start dismissing your contribution?

While I am regularly the first in the queue to criticise the current peer review system. I am also very grateful that publication represents a line in the sand under which I won't have to continue working on a project. In a world in which I had continually documented every step of every experiment, I can imagine that it is potentially possible to find a *post hoc* defence for every step in a protocol. But the painstaking nature and time involved in going through old work would be an added burden that I cannot welcome with any enthusiasm. Personally, in a world when I have the option of working on a new project or endlessly and repeatedly defending old ones, I'd pick the new project every time.

10.9   Are preprints published?

As they each have a DOI (Digital Object Identifier), they are in their own way already published.

Another point is that these articles are picking up citations. And there is a new concern that these articles are being cited, even when they are subsequently available through a published journal. This is one of my personal concerns with using a preprint service. I'm happy to put the paper out there for public comment, but the idea that it'll remain there and that readers won't necessarily be redirected to the peer-reviewed version does concern me.

Another question is what happens to manuscripts that are placed on preprint servers, and are then sent out for review but not published because they are fundamentally flawed? It's not as if the reviews are not made, but there is no automatic link to the reviews by the journal that conducted them.

There are certainly a lot of manuscripts out there with fundamental flaws. These are often sent for peer review, but those reviews pointing out the errors won't necessarily make it back to the comments page on the preprint server. I think that this is a serious problem. The reviewers have spent time and effort and the very reason they do this is so that manuscripts with fundamental flaws don't find their way into the literature. However, preprint servers have, perhaps unwittingly, found a loophole that allows manuscripts that are not scientifically robust a backdoor to citations.

If preprints are fundamentally flawed, can't everyone spot it?

No. Reviewers are chosen by an editor with great care because of their speciality area is in their particular domain. They have insights that not everyone will be aware of and these are an important aspect of the purpose of peer review.

I edit for the journal *PeerJ* (www.peerj.com). Although there can be various reasons to be rejected from *PeerJ*, normally it means that your paper is not scientifically sound. As *PeerJ* has no selection for impact, rejection does not normally mean that it can be simply submitted to another journal. I have noticed that manuscripts that I have rejected from *PeerJ* are still available as preprints without any comment on their failure during peer review. In my opinion, this is not good as it essentially ignores the input given by both reviewers and editors. The article appears as if they have had no comments or attention, when this is not the case. In a system where we move to relying more on preprints, why would we want to ignore chosen peer reviewers for whom this article was within their specialist area? According to Google Scholar, the rejected articles are gaining citations, again raising concerns that rejection by peer review is not a hurdle to entering the scientific literature. All of this calls for reviews to be linked more directly to preprints, no matter where they are published. A model that deals directly with this is overlay journals.

10.10   The exciting new world of Overlay Journals

Having said that preprints won't replace the role of peer review, what if we did have good, editorially coordinated peer review of preprints? What if, instead of these manuscripts effectively leaving the preprint system, they were updated together with the reviews that prompted the updates, each with their own linked DOI? What if the journals themselves were simply pointing to collections of papers that had been curated in this way? Simply a website that throws a veneer of a journal as waypoints to peer reviewed articles. This world has already been imagined and is functioning in mathematics, where Overlay Journals have begun to prosper.

According to Brown (2010), the idea of overlaying has been with us for some time, and exists as websites that offer a series of links to other papers. In this way, a review article could be considered an 'overlay paper', the contents of Web of Science as an 'overlay database'. But, for me at least, this is not where the real potential lies. Instead, imagine the overlay journal as a way in which academics entirely remove the need for publishers. The need for this is increasingly evident as we become more familiar with the ways in which we rely on traditional publishing models to pervade our scientific project with confirmation bias. Overlay journals no longer require a publisher to store the publication. This is done at the preprint server. The reviews are housed at the same *arXiv* site (or would be in an ideal and transparent version Rittman, 2020), as is the manuscript in its final form after being accepted by the overlay journal editor. The authors themselves are responsible for the final layout. The Overlay Journal co-ordinates the reviews and conducts the editorial work, and then simply acts as a pointer to the finished product: no papers, no publishers, no editorial management software, no costs and all papers are Diamond OA!

The journal *Discrete Analysis* (discreteanalysisjournal.com) (indexed in both Web of Science and Scopus) was the first of these new '*arXiv* overlay journals' (since 2017), and visiting their website will allow you to quickly appreciate what an Overlay Journal is. Each 'published' paper still sits on its original preprint server. The overlay journal itself offers a brief editorial summary of what you'll find if you click through to the paper. This is a fantastic idea in that it pitches editors back into being responsible content curators. As an editor I'd want to be motivated to publish a paper that I liked in order to write an editorial summary about it.

Because only the accepted version is provided with an 'article number' and the style file of the journal layout, the author then produces the final version of record (VoR) of the accepted manuscript by running the style file with LaTeX. All of this is possible with free software, for example by using R Markdown (Xie et al., 2018).

Using preprint servers also allows the entire process to be transparent, very quickly becoming associated with other great initiatives like the Centre for Open Science – OSF (www.cos.io).

10.10.1 What do traditional publishers think of 'Overlay Journals'?

Surely, the onset of 'Overlay Journals' should have publishers quaking in their boots? Strangley not. But their response should really be enough to wake us up.

"They're probably only going to succeed in disciplines where a no-frills approach to publishing is acceptable... I think that the real threat to our traditional model... is if Overlay Journals have **Impact Factors** and can provide the same services, and they are free... then I think that that does pose a threat."

—Claire Rawlinson, Highwire Press Inc. 2017[1]

As this has already happened (for the journal *Discrete Analysis*), it would be interesting to know how traditional publishers are going to prevent an Overlay Journal take-over.

10.10.2 What is happening in Biological Sciences?

One of the original electronic journals, *Journal of Medical Internet Research* (JMIR; www.jmir.org), announced in 2019 that it will launch an overlay journal covering biology, a so-called 'superjournal', *JMIRx* (Eysenbach, 2019). This overlay journal operates by editors choosing preprints that they want to publish ('editorial prospecting'), and then approaching authors and reviewers, and also by authors pitching their preprints to the editors. Today *JMIRx/Bio* (bio.jmirx.org) accepts any preprint published on *bioRxiv*. Although *JMIRx/Bio*, and sister journal *JMRIx/Psy* (psy.jmirx.org), were launched in 2020, I cannot find any articles submitted (by mid-2021). The sister journal *JMIRx/Med* (med.jmirx.org) launched at the same time and in the same area as other JMIR journals, and has a rapidly expanding publication base.

Another preprint led service is *F1000Research* (f1000research.com), which grew (via a buy out by Taylor & Francis) from the peer recommendation site Faculty Opinions (facultyopinions.com). *F1000Research* requires preprint submission on their server, and then co-ordinates postprint peer review which

---

[1]https://youtu.be/ADecAXLrKoA

is all accessible online in the same location. Like other Gold OA journals, *F1000Research* charges an impressive Article Processing Charge (APC), and does not aspire to an Impact Factor.

There's an excellent tie-in here with transparency. Because preprints are Diamond OA and reviews are OA, the process is all transparent.

A nearly 'overlay' model is *Peer Community in Evolutionary Biology* (*PCI-Evol Biol*: evolbiol.peercommunityin.org/), launched in January 2017. This comes very close to the '*arXiv* Overlay Journal' model described above. These preprints are submitted to *PCI-Evol Biol*, and are reviewed and (if they aren't rejected), a recommendation is given. The site then publishes the recommendation from peers as well as pointing to the preprint. However, unlike *Discrete Analysis*, the preprint remains 'unpublished' despite the peer review and can then be taken onto a traditional journal or (since 2021) be published in their own journal *Peer Community Journal*. There is a growing list of journals whose editors will accept recommendations from *PCI-EvolBiol*, and may use the reviews when appropriate. However, it's also worth noting that there are a small number of journals that will not accept preprints recommended by *PCI-EvolBiol*. While *Peer Community in Evolutionary Biology* does not publish their peer reviewed articles, another initiative from *Peer Community In* takes a step backwards to get a step closer (see below).

The journal *eLife* is also taking steps towards becoming an Overlay Journal, with their implementation of a **preprint only** submission route (Eisen et al., 2020). Although *eLife* appears to embrace all the advantages of transparency in their use of preprints, there is still a significant barrier that has recently jumped from USD 2500 to 3000 for the privilege to publish (*eLife* has an APC waiver system which is not seen by editors). Again the question of what exactly scholars are paying such high fees for comes to the forefront.

10.10.3   Preregistration and a commitment to publish

Registering your proposal (or any research plan), means that you can present a historical document to a journal (probably four to five years later) to show that you have tested the hypotheses that you originally intended to. This is simply a way of being transparent in your science, and enables you to demonstrate that you have not been P hacking or HARKing. Similarly, you can demonstrate that you are not 'salami-slicing' your results. Moreover, there is some evidence to suggest that reviews of preregistered research plans inhibit researchers from leveraging their own beliefs to generate the kind of surprising results we associate with high Impact Factors (Gross and Bergstrom, 2021).

Another initiative from *Peer Community In* is the possibility of submitting to their Registered Reports, which goes much further towards removing the confirmation bias. The Registered Report (RR) is in effect the registration of a proposal (i.e. preregistration) with review. If the RR is approved by reviewers then the study is, in principle, given the green light for publication whether or not the hypothesis posed is accepted or rejected. I say 'in principle' because those same reviewers are shown the manuscript again once the results are in. They need to check that the methods proposed were followed, the analyses were conducted in the same way they were proposed, and that the conclusions are justified by the results. Peer Community In are offering to organise the two sets of peer review. In addition, there are a bunch of journals that have already signed up to accept RRs that are signed off after completion (notable among these is *PeerJ*). To me, this represents an important step in the right direction towards transparency and the elimination of confirmation bias. What would be great to see is the number of conventional journals sign up with RRs based on the quality of the study design and execution, and the concomitant abandonment of Impact Factor as a driving force in publishing.

10.10.4   Choose non-profit preprint servers

Preprint servers have the potential to take away traditional publishers' business. For this reason, you will see that some publishers have launched their own preprint services. However, there are plenty of preprint servers that have nothing to do with publishers, including the most ubiquitous. These are non-profit transparent organisations, and we all have an interest in them staying that way. Instead use Open Source Tools and transparent resources (Kramer and Bosman 2016).

10.11   Peeriodicals – another twist on the idea of an Overlay Journal

The launch in 2018 of *Peeriodicals* (peeriodicals.com) puts another twist on the idea of an Overlay Journal. This time, the *Peeriodical* is a site where anyone puts together a collection of any published papers or pre-prints that they curate themselves on a topic. They don't pass them out for any further review, but they are in effect another kind of curated Overlay.

10.12   Should you submit your manuscript as a preprint?

Here are some reasons for and against submitting your manuscript as a preprint:

10.12.1   For

- Your manuscript needs to be cited by another paper that you are submitting and you are worried that the peer review process will take too long.
  - This is especially appropriate in the need to be transparent to demonstrate that you are not 'salami slicing' your work.
- You are applying for a scholarship, a grant or job and want to be able to show that you have a body of work that is ready to be published, even if it is not formally published yet. Using preprints, you can allow the hiring committee or potential employer access to your work. This is really much more impressive than claiming manuscripts are 'in preparation' on your CV.
- You are presenting some unpublished work at a conference and you want people to be able to access it (e.g. through scanning a QR code)
- You are submitting a grant application and want to demonstrate that you have sufficient data, although it isn't yet published
- You are aware that another lab is working on a similar project and are worried that submitting to peer review will scoop your findings.
- Your work has immediacy that it might not have after (potentially) 3 months of peer review. It may be that by releasing your preprint you can contribute to an ongoing debate that otherwise you'll potentially miss.
- It's free. No APC or other fees are involved with depositing your preprint.
- You have the potential to increase your network when people you have never met read your work.
- You are concerned that you've missed something important or perhaps analysed something in a novel way that others might be able to help with. You want this chance at feedback before submitting to peer review.
- Your manuscript crashed out of peer review with comments that you felt were unfair or unsubstantiated. You are looking for more balanced comments.

- In the above case, you might be able to use your preprint as leverage to persuade an editor that your contribution should be fast tracked into their journal.

- If you can generate enough buzz and positive feedback, you might be able to get leverage on an editor for submission to a journal with a higher Impact Factor.

- You have a working group that you actively want to share your publication with, even before it is published.

- This is the only submission route for 'Overlay Journals'
  - Peer Community Journal (peercommunityjournal.org)
  - PCI-Evol Biol in Biological Sciences
  - JMIRx|Bio accepts any preprint published on *bioRxiv* since 2020

- This is the only submission route for some other journals (e.g. *eLife*: Eisen et al., 2020).

10.12.2 Against

- Any of your co-authors don't want the manuscript submitted as a preprint before peer review.
- You feel that public access might mean that your results are misinterpreted, this should be on you to get it right before you submit it (especially in public health).
- There is a real chance that others can use the access to your work and publish it before you.
  - It's worth adding here that while you might believe that there are lots of people out there who might want to steal your work, this is a general paranoia that is very common in early career researchers. Few fields in Biological Sciences really have valid examples of data theft or idea theft.
- Preprints are another example of how everything is too rushed these days.
  - I've heard this opinion, but wonder why these authors wouldn't simply hold onto their manuscript until they feel that it's ready.

I can't really come up with a lot of reasons against submitting a preprint (I've had to add some I have heard other people saying). This is possibly because I'm broadly in favour of preprints and see that there is value there. However, I've done it with only a fraction of papers submitted in the last 5 years. Why?

My experience of preprints, in terms of feedback and reviews, is disappointing. Although these get widely shared on social media, and garner a large number of downloads, they don't generate comments from colleagues. Even when we have sent links of preprints to colleagues asking directly for feedback, we've received little to nothing. This does not mean that preprints are worthless. I think that they have great potential, and they may work better for you in your field than for me in mine. Moreover, preprint servers now hold the potential to free academics from the tyranny of profit hungry publishing houses.

At this point, I should say that I have not (yet) made any public comments on a preprint. When I have looked at preprints, I (generally) have downloaded them in order to look at some of the details (often the methods or analyses), when there's a dearth of peer reviewed (published) material. There are a few references to preprints in this book. I'll replace them if I find that they have been published. But what should I do if the published version doesn't contain the point that I'm citing on? In this case, I'll delete the citation and no longer make the claim because there is the chance that the result did not stand up to the rigours of peer review.

Part II

Publishing your work

11

Writing your cover letter

Many journals require that you write a cover letter to the editor on submission. Each journal should tell you what this letter should contain. This will vary from journal to journal as some may have a set of check boxes that cover some points in their editorial management software, while others may want a written declaration. It is very important that your letter contains all of the information required by the journal. If not, it could lead to an automated desk rejection.

Some journals have a text box in their submission software for you to paste the text of this letter. If there is a text box, then I suggest that you do not compose it on the fly, but plan it out and write it in a word processor so that you can catch any silly spelling or grammatical errors. Other journals might expect you to upload a pdf letter on headed paper from your institution. Make sure you know what is required and that you are prepared. The reason for a formal signed letter on headed paper is that in some submissions, this letter is used as a legal declaration.

Your cover letter is a professional, formal letter, and should be written as such. Use the conventional letter writing format, including addresses, date, signature, etc. If you are unsure what this looks like, there is some great advice on the web, including templates to use.

Address your letter to the journal editor. One of the nice things about academic titles is that they are gender neutral, so use them: **Dear Dr. Jones**, or **Dear Prof. Smith**. Even if this person has an office down the hall and you see them every day, keep the cover letter professional. It will go on file with the publisher.

The following points should be covered (where relevant) in the order given as a default. Any content and style requests from the journal, about how the cover letter should be written, clearly takes precedent.

1. The title of your manuscript, the type of submission (review, research article, letter, etc.) and the name of the journal that you are submitting to. Note that it is all too easy to forget to change the journal name when you are submitting to another journal. In my time as editor, I've seen some very nice letters explaining how the

DOI: 10.1201/9781003220886-11

manuscript is appropriate to a completely different journal. Not a good start!

2. Statement that your manuscript has not been published or submitted elsewhere, and that all authors have approved the submission. There are other statements that are required by certain journals, and sometimes the journal requests that you copy and paste their text as the cover letter is kept and used as a legal declaration. Also it may include information about ethics clearance and any permits required having been obtained and available should the paper be accepted. Note that you don't need to include all of this information unless the journal that you are submitting to requires it.

3. Include information about why your research is suitable to the scope the journal that you have submitted it to. This requires you to have checked the scope of the journal itself and have thought about exactly how your paper aligns to this. Bear in mind that this is a real problem. Editors get far too many papers that do not fit the scope of their journal, and it takes time to process and reject these (so they are not appreciated).

4. Novel and innovative research. For journals where the Impact Factor is important, you may want to emphasise what is novel about your study, and therefore in the minds of the editors deserving of the impact.

5. Important information that the editor must know. For example, if the manuscript was previously rejected with an invitation to resubmit (then also include the manuscript number that was given previously). Or (rarely) if you (or others) have previously retracted a similar study, with reasons why this manuscript is not affected.

6. Connections to other ongoing research. If relevant, state what other manuscripts are already submitted to this or other journals. For example, is your work part of an ongoing consortium or research programme? The idea here is to demonstrate to the editor that your manuscript will be cited in a timely manor.

7. A final brief statement to the effect that: **'We declare that we have no conflicts of interest'.** Unless of course you do, then state succinctly what it is.

11.1 Do editors read cover letters?

This is a moot point in that you will never know. Some editors definitely read every cover letter (Kenar, 2016). Even new journals have retained the need for a cover letter when they have stripped down the submission process to a minimum (e.g. *eLife*), and so my suggestion is that it is needed and, hopefully, it will be read. However, every editor at every journal is likely to have their own method of what they regard as important to read (Moustafa, 2015), with many actively trying to minimise this. Where there are legal requirements, it's not likely that editors will read them, but editorial managers may well make sure that these are present in order not to get a pre-review (desk) rejection.

Chief editors may read parts of the cover letter along with the abstract before deciding which Associate Editor should be assigned. Some chief editors will even leave this to the Associate Editor. The Associate Editor should read your cover letter in full, together with the metadata and other salient information therein. They should also read the entire manuscript. It is worth noting that reviewers are not given access to cover letters.

11.2 What not to do in your cover letter

- Try not to make your cover letter too long. A single page should be enough to cover all of the points above.
- Don't copy and paste your abstract. There will be a place for this in the metadata on the submissions site.
- Avoid specialist terms that the editor may not know.
- Don't try and oversell your study, or make excessive claims.
- Avoid 'first ever' claims, as they won't impress the editor.
- Don't suggest potential reviewers unless the journal rubric specifically requests this in the cover letter.
- Similarly, don't suggest people that you don't want to review your article, or start any history of why your submission is complicated by third parties.
- Don't deviate from a formal letter style.
- Don't have spelling and grammatical errors.
- Avoid formatting the letter in a way that might make it difficult to read:
  - Don't be tempted to reduce font size to get more in (keep to Ariel 11 point)
  - If you need more space to keep your letter to 1 page, change the margin sizes
  - Don't fully justify text (left justify only)
  - If you are recycling your letter, check that you have changed **everything**.

12

Suggesting reviewers

You will often be asked to suggest reviewers as you submit your manuscript. This can be part of your cover letter, or data that you need to fill in during the submission process. Keep in mind that supplying a name alone will not be considered sufficient, you will need their name, the name of their institution and their email address. Some journals will not accept addresses that do not come from institutions unless they can be verified. The reason for this is that there has been an outbreak of fraudulent reviewers, where authors suggested fake reviewers or gave email addresses that they manufactured (see Brainard and You, 2018).

In keeping with the spirit of peer review, you should suggest people that you think will provide insightful reviews. These could be people that work in the same area (but that aren't involved in your study). Personally, I name the same set of people that I would invite myself if I were editing. People that I believe would provide a constructive and unbiased review.

12.1 Who should you not suggest?

- Anyone who is an author or in the acknowledgements
- Anyone else you feel may have a conflict of interest
    - connected with the work but not an author
    - someone who was on your review committee
- Someone in your department or even at your institution (there may be exceptions here, but often journals will not consider people with matching institutional emails)
- Friends, labmates or even relatives (even if you genuinely think that they would do a good job)
- People who are regular co-authors (grant panels specifically ban you from naming these people as potential reviewers. If you have a large network, this can be problematic).

DOI: 10.1201/9781003220886-12

12.2   Who should you oppose?

In addition to allowing you to suggest reviewers, many journals allow you to oppose reviewers. I usually leave this blank. If you have a particular lab or persons who you suspect will not follow the spirit of peer review, you could enter them here.

12.3   Who will the editor use?

It is worth bearing in mind that whoever you suggest, the editor may not use them. I have talked to editors who will never consider anyone recommended by authors as a matter of course, because they assume that these people will be positively biased towards the authors. This same editor said that they'd always use at least one of the opposed reviewers. This rarely fits with journal policy.

As an editor, I will often use one of the reviewers suggested by the authors if they fit my (following) criteria. I will make sure that I balance this with another reviewer or two not suggested by the authors. To select reviewers, I will read the submission and look for citations of similar studies, or techniques (depending on the type of paper). From the citations, I will find the paper (preferably published in the last 3 years) and use the corresponding author's address. I will also try to visit the website of the senior (last) author to see whether they have a lab that is still active in this area, and especially I will be looking for post-docs or Early Career Scientists who cover the same topic. If they are there, I will invite them. If not, I will write to the lab head in the hope that they may well recommend one of their post-docs. This process can take a long time, especially hunting down email addresses that constantly bounce back from the journal's editorial manager software.

I will also use people that I know in my own network, especially an extended network. People whose conference talks I've seen or other papers in my area that I have read or cited myself. I try not to bombard my own close network too much with demands for reviews. I try not to use reviewers auto-suggested by editorial management software. In my experience, these are not suitable people. Whether this is the same for other editors, I cannot say.

If the manuscript is a resubmission, I will try to use the same reviewers that made previous reviews. This isn't always possible, and I know that it is a source of upset for authors when they receive new reviews on a second or even third round of review. I don't think that any editors will do this deliberately, but reviewers do have the option of indicating that they are not willing to reread a resubmission. If this is the case for most or all of the reviewers, then you are likely to face an entirely fresh round of peer review.

13

Choosing the right journal

In this section I provide steps to go from a potentially very long list of journals where you might publish, to choosing the one where you will submit your manuscript first. As you work through the steps, keep notes on why you exclude journals at each step. You may want to revisit these criteria later, or explain to your co-authors why a particular journal was not considered.

Although your article can be found from anyone outside of the normal journal readership, it is important to publish your paper in the correct journal for your study for the following reasons:

- The editor will desk reject your manuscript if it is not appropriate (and you'll waste their time).
- Many reviewers give feedback tailored to the journal, and this will not be appropriate in the wrong journal.
- Perhaps most importantly, you are likely to get additional readers in the correct journal that might not find your paper otherwise.
- Note that there are no Impact Factor journals for which the above is not relevant, and these are discussed separately.

This section is geared towards the 'current' model in the life sciences of journal title as a measure of quality. The reality is that this model is shifting, and we may well end up with another (better) open model in the future based around preprint servers and overlay journals. The current reliance on journal titles is driving a toxic culture in Biological Sciences that is becoming increasingly recognised, even by those who are gatekeepers for this model (see Part IV). To reflect this viewpoint, and help drive a culture of change, I have placed Impact Factor outside of this list of steps. In doing so, I acknowledge that you and your co-authors may well be operating inside the current publisher driven model advocating for Impact Factor as a step with high priority. Even if this is your reality, I hope that you will acknowledge and appreciate that this is not the way that journals should be chosen.

As an Early Career Researcher, you are likely to need to think of review, promotion and tenure when considering where to publish. An important point to be aware of is how your institution perceives quality, prestige and impact. These are rather nebulous terms that can sometimes be well defined by institutions, but faculty often mix-up these terms and frequently rely on Impact Factor to define them (Morales et al., 2021). You should, therefore, consult documentation on review, promotion and tenure at your institution, and/or consult your mentor. You may then want to add these definitions at the top of your table in your journal selection process.

I'm going to suggest that you keep a spreadsheet with the answers to the steps below as columns, and different journals as rows. If your submission is rejected from the first journal choice, you can then use this spreadsheet so that you know where to submit next (i.e. just do the work once). This spreadsheet may well come in handy for future similar submissions.

13.0.1   Indexing

You want other people to be able to find the work that you publish, and so selecting a journal that is already indexed in one of the major literature databases (e.g. Web of Science or Scopus) is important. Be aware that when new journals are indexed, they are usually done with their entire back catalogue. Thus, if a journal advertises that it will be listed by one of major literature databases, your submission will likely be listed eventually, even if not immediately.

13.0.2   The subject area

No matter what your paper is about it will fall within an existing subject area. A good way of determining your subject area is to look at those listed by literature database like Web of Science or Scopus. These databases have subject areas which contain groups of journals. You can look through the journals that you cite in your references, then check with Web of Science or Scopus to see which subject area the majority of them are grouped into.

Journals have different hierarchies of scope. Some journals attempt to take on the full gambit of science (e.g. *Science* and *Nature*) while others are only interested in a particular taxonomic group. In general, the Impact Factor of the journal is likely to be linked to the diversity of the scope. This is not always the case. There are some taxonomically specific journals with high Impact Factors, and there are some general journals with low Impact Factors.

Once you have determined your subject area make a list of the journals within this area. Based on your reading of literature pertinent to your manuscript, try to decide whether your manuscript is likely to be accepted by a journal with a high rank. Many databases rank journals into quartiles (Q1 to Q4), and these can be useful groups to set your aims at. Note that these will change depending on the literature database that your institution uses.

13.0.3 The journal scope and readership

Every journal has a scope that is stated on their website. Your manuscript must fit into the scope of the journal that you select. In order to get your candidate list of journals you now need to visit their websites to look at their scope in detail. Ill fitting scope is the most common cause of a desk rejection (Schimel et al., 2014; Teixeira da Silva et al., 2018). Journal Scope is also most strongly aligned to readership, that is the specific readership that you want to reach when publishing your article. Readership was recognised as the strongest factor for North American faculty in selecting a journal (Niles et al., 2020).

If your potential journal list is long, I suggest that you lead with the journals whose articles you have already cited in your manuscript. In the journals that you enter into your spreadsheet, quickly summarise the scopes of your choice journals and make some notes on how your manuscript fits them. This will help when writing your cover letter.

13.0.4 Ownership of the content

In this book, I have made a plea for the movement to an Open publishing model. Note that your choice of journal will dictate who ends up owning the content: i.e. copyright. Most for-profit publishers insist on owning the content of the journals that they publish. This means that if you ever want to use the content that you created (such as a figure in a book), then you will need to approach those publishers for permission. Traditionally, for-profit publishers have retained copyright on their content as this makes for another potential income stream for the future (think text books that use graphs from journal papers). In the case of society owned journals, the copyright can be retained by the society. Most Open Access publishers have been forced into a Rights Retention Strategy by cOAlition S, and consequently, this should be a general trend in all journals: copyright is retained by the authors with a Creative Commons licence. If you want to know more about what the different Creative Commons licences mean, they have a very good explanation on their website: creativecommons.org

Although I've listed ownership of content as Step 4 in this scheme, I would suggest to you that it is not incompatible with any journal. As owner of your content, you have the right to archiving your Green OA wherever you please. Wherever you publish, make sure that you retain ownership of your content, and if this is not the case, then insist that you want to retain the right to your own content once your article is accepted. Think of it from the other side of the desk: if the author wrote to you as editor and said that they want to retain ownership of their content – on what grounds do you (as editor) have to refuse them? Owning your own content seems like a trivial step in the massive movement from closed to open science, but it is a very significant step forward that all scientists should own their content.

13.0.5   Current contents

Now that you have a shorter list, it's time for you to look at the current contents of the journals that are on their website. The contents for the last two years should reflect the policy of the current editor for accepting manuscripts. You should be looking for papers that look similar to your manuscript in their scope.

If you see papers that look directly comparable to your own then make a note of what they are. Your list of journals should now be less than ten.

13.0.6   Society journals

Academic publishing started with society journals, and I think that they are still worth supporting if you can. You or your co-authors may be members of particular academic societies, and may have a preference therefore to publish in their society's journal. See below for other potential advantages of publishing in a society journal.

13.0.7   Transparent credibility

Transparency in science is very important and should be part and parcel of your own work. When you have made a real effort to be transparent, you should look for journals that do the same. There is a badge system used for transparency in science. See Kidwell et al. (2016), or see Marshall and Strine (2021), for an example of how this can be applied.

13.0.8   Knowing the journal from the inside

Your mentor or co-authors could be an Editor or Associate Editor (past or present) of one of your target journals. Or there may be someone in your department or institute that you could consult. I am not suggesting that you use their influence to help you get published, this conflict of interest is strictly prohibited by most journals. Instead, these people can help you decide whether or not your submission will be welcomed or desk rejected.

Reject without review is typical for manuscripts whose authors have not followed steps 2 to 4. It can still happen, even if you have. Reject without review is such a waste of everybody's time that you should avoid it if at all possible.

13.0.9   Is there a special issue?

Special issues are a great way for your work to get better exposure, both to others that are participating in the special issue, and to those who come across the entire issue later (see Part I).

13.0.10   Avoiding the predators

You must make sure that the journal you plan to submit to is not a predatory journal. Follow the check list in Part IV.

13.0.11   Financial considerations to publishing

Check for the journal APC and whether you or your institution will be able to pay. In an ideal world, there wouldn't be any more barriers to you publishing your contribution to the collective of scientific knowledge. Not only is it not an ideal world, but I would argue that there has never been a less ideal time for publishing science. Read more on this later in the book.

13.0.12   Type of peer review

Another factor that may influence your choice of where to publish is the type of reviewing done by each journal. These reviewer flavours are discussed in detail in part 1.

13.0.13   Time to first decision

Sometimes you will be in a hurry to publish, and journals have different mean times to first decision. In general, this is driven by the responsiveness of the editorial team. Some journals, with fast turnaround times, advertise their time to first decision and so this may influence your decision about whether or not to publish there. Remember that if you are desperate to get a manuscript out into the public domain, you can always submit a preprint.

13.0.14   Open Access

Some journals are exclusively Open Access (OA) meaning that you will need to pay (unless they are Diamond OA) in order to publish your accepted manuscript (author pays). Different types of OA are covered in a subsequent chapter (see Part II). More information on OA is provided in Part IV, and I encourage you to read this before you decide to pay any research money towards OA publishing Article Processing Charges (APCs).

Your university may have a deal with some OA publishers (especially if you are based at a European institution) so it's well worth making a note of this. If in doubt, talk to your librarian. However, watch out for manipulative publisher deals that make you more likely to publish OA when your institution has a 'read-and-publish' or 'transformative' deal. Remember to ask yourself your motivation for why you are choosing your journal. Morally, choice by publishing company should never be high up on anyone's list.

13.0.15   Page charges

Note that some journals that remain behind paywalls still demand page charges. These can be quite substantial if you come from a lab with no money for page charges. In my experience American society journals regularly have page charges. These may well be reduced for members, or you may be eligible for a page charge fee waiver.

13.0.16   Fee waiver

Note that with all of the above you may be eligible for a waiver to page charges or Open Access fees. Who gets a waiver will be discussed later in the book.

13.0.17   Impact Factor

The Impact Factor of the journal may be an important motivation in your choice, or that of your advisor. I've left it off my list of stepwise criteria as I hope that it's not going to influence you according to the San Francisco Declaration on Research Assessment (known as DORA). If Impact Factor is important to you, include it in the list that you produce and make a note of the most recent Impact Factor for each journal. There's more about the Impact Factor in another chapter.

13.0.18   No Impact Factor journal

In this book I refer to journals that have no interest in their Impact Factor as 'no Impact Factor'. Of course, if these journals are listed by Impact Factor providing databases (and most are), then they will have an Impact Factor and this can be high – even higher than other journals that attempt to inflate their Impact Factors (see Part IV). Instead, what I mean is that these journals are operating at minimum standards of technical soundness (so-called 'negative selection'), instead of the AKP (Anna Karenina Principle) selection of only papers that are thought by their gatekeepers to uphold or increase the journal IF.

There's no problem to publish in a journal that has no interest in Impact Factor. Indeed, it can be seen as 'the right thing to do', with respect to confirmation bias. This is the way that all science was published prior to the dominance of citation metrics. If you are submitting to a 'no Impact Factor journal' then you should be aware that this is what their speciality is: an emphasis on the technical soundness, rather than whether or not a significant result was found. You need to be aware as this is how inclusion of such publications in your CV will be regarded by peers. The list of 'no Impact Factor journals' is growing, and they tend to be online only, Gold OA and carry substantial article processing charges.

13.1   Shortlist

Once you have your shortlist of journals to consider, take it to your mentor. Together with your co-authors rework your list into something that you all agree with. Rank your list by journals that you want to try first and those that are your last options at the end.

Keep the list so that if you are rejected by the first journal on your list you know where you're going to next.

14

Open Access or a paywall for your manuscript?

There are many well established benefits to publishing an Open Access (OA) paper where there is no paywall to any readers. These include increased citations, increased exposure and coverage by the media, not to mention increased interactions with the public and the moral and ethical duty to be able to share research as widely as possible. Many studies are now suggesting that the advantages go even deeper (see a collection of studies curated by Tennant, 2017). However the current reality is that most publishers will then require you to pay in order to produce your publication open access. There are chapters later on in this book that discuss the importance of open access. In this chapter, I review the different OA models available. At this period in time, the names are somewhat fluid, and you may not find the specific term mentioned here on the publishers' website.

14.1 Closed Access: i.e. The Paywall

This refers to the need for your institution or you personally to be subscribed to the journal in order to access the content. This is the traditional model in academic publishing. If you are a member of an academic society then you may get access to their society journals through your membership. This is still effectively a paywall that is maintained by the publisher and the society together (Figure 14.1).

It is sometimes hard to know if there is a paywall if your university subscribes to the publisher or the journal that you are interested in. There has been a lot of headway made in having seamless integration and access to articles behind paywalls from within university IP addresses.

If you try working from home then you will quickly find out which journals exist behind paywalls. There is another chapter with ideas on how to get around the paywall if you need to.

Although publishing an article behind a paywall is often frowned upon these days it usually means that there'll be no cost for you as the author, and so for

DOI: 10.1201/9781003220886-14

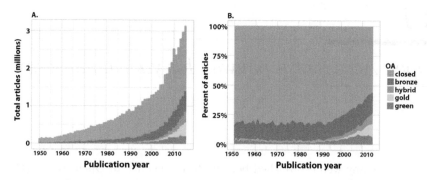

FIGURE 14.1: The majority of publications still sit behind a paywall.
Figure 2 redrawn from Piwowar et al. (2018) shows the increasing number (A)
and proportion (B) of a random sample of 100,000 papers published with a
CrossRef DOI with an increasing trend in Gold and Hybrid OA publications
since 2005. This figure does not represent the Grey and Black OA content.
Note that reproduction of published material is possible if it is published under
CC BY.

many academics this is still the only real option in terms of publishing their
scholarly work in an academic journal.

There follows a brief description of each of the OA models. See Piwowar et al.
(2018) for a historical review of these different models:

14.2 Open Access (OA)

There is a bewildering array of different Open Access types. Entries in the list
below are not mutually exclusive. Moreover, you may not be aware how your
manuscript may be treated, and it is not always possible to predict the level
of OA your article will be published with in many journals. Each journal will
likely have their own policy, tied to the publisher in many cases.

14.2.1 Gratis OA

Gratis OA simply refers to the ability for anyone to access the text free, and
without any paywall.

14.2.2 Libre OA

Some definitions of OA extend beyond simply being allowed to access the text for free (Gratis OA) to it bearing a license so that you can share, redistribute and reuse (Libre OA). With Libre OA everyone is able to share, redistribute or copy the content. The Creative Commons (CC-BY 4.0) licence allows others to 'remix, transform, and build upon the material for any purpose, even commercially'.

A good example of this is my ability to publish Figure 14.1 from Piwowar et al. (2018) as the content of *PeerJ* is published under CC BY licence.

14.2.3 Green OA

This is an option no matter what journal you publish in, including closed journals behind the paywall. The accepted manuscript, before it has been typeset, is deposited in your institutional repository; usually your library hosts this. This is sometimes referred to as a **postprint** (manuscript with changes made following peer review) – the same version that has been accepted by the journal. Once your paper is published by the journal, anyone can access the manuscript that was accepted because it is available free from your institutional repository. However the typeset paper will remain behind the publishers' paywall (i.e. closed). Note that this version will not be the Version of Record, it may be that some of the text will change with copy editing. However, for people who want Open Access to your work, this Green OA version should suffice.

When you deposit your author version to your institutional repository, make sure that you add a Creative Commons Attribution (creativecommons.org) license (CC BY). In theory, this turns your work into something that is Libre Open Access. Although the wording will be the same in the Closed OA version eventually available from the publisher, the prior attribution of CC BY to your Green OA work should mean that all subsequent versions are Libre OA. There are a number of reasons why this may not be the case, and you should be aware of two of these (Khoo, 2021). First are your obligations to your funders. For example, your funders may have specific requirements about how you publish, and a prior rights attribution may conflict. Funders may have other restrictions on your publishing including embargo periods. With many publishers you may be required to sign an acceptance letter that specifically states that it supersedes any previous licensing commitments including self archiving copies that you make CC BY. Your previous CC BY commitments to your pre-print may then place you in a legal conflict. Publishers are unlikely to assert their license unless you try to assert yours.

If you are unsure about whether or not to deposit a copy in your institutional repository and what license should be attributed to this, then ask your librarian.

You may need to furnish them with details of your funding and the journal where your manuscript has been accepted for publication.

14.2.4 Bronze OA

Bronze Open Access is an option at the discretion of the publishers. Only some publishers do this for some of their content. For example, they may decide that a certain thematic issue should be open access, an editorial, or review article. There is some debate about whether this bronze model is truly OA as it often still carries copyright restrictions.

14.2.5 Delayed OA

Some journals choose to have their archived content available for all readers without a paywall. This could be after two or five years. Like Bronze OA, there is some debate about whether delayed OA is truly open as it often still carries the publishers' copyright restrictions.

14.2.6 Gold OA

In a journal with gold open access it is compulsory for you to pay the open access fee (or Article Processing Charge, often referred to as APC) in order to publish your paper. These APCs can be very large, often more than USD 1000 (see Part IV). If your choice of journal is gold open access, then make sure you know where the fees are coming from. The history of Gold OA is an interesting one that you can read in Part IV.

Examples of gold open access journals are *PLOS ONE*, *F1000Research* and *PeerJ*, and an increasing hoard of 'no Impact Factor' journals. The advantage to these journals is that as soon as you publish your work in them, everyone will have access to it without any paywall. The disadvantage is that you may not be able to afford to publish there. The disadvantages of these journals are now becoming very prominent in the Biological Sciences, such that you may be excluded from increasing numbers of journals in your field. Alarmingly, journals with higher Impact Factors are also charging ever increasing sums to publish Gold OA (Gray, 2020). Gray (2020) makes the important point that prestige (often confused with Impact Factor) is being allocated a higher price in Gold OA, that is likely to disadvantage and disenfranchise scientists from less wealthy institutions and countries. This is likely to reinforce an increasing dichotomy between rich and poor researchers. We will take another look at who pays for OA later in the book.

Watch out for predatory journals among those journals with Gold OA. Predatory publication will be discussed in full later.

14.2.7   Hybrid OA

Hybrid OA journals are increasingly the norm. You can decide upon acceptance of your manuscript whether or not you want to pay the fee to make your article open access. Again, note that your institution may have a deal with the publisher which means that anything you publish there is open access. It is well worth knowing these things in advance before you submit. If you can't afford to pay the open access fee then your manuscript will remain behind a paywall and be only available to subscribers.

Note that many journals refer to paying for OA inside a hybrid journal as 'Gold OA'. Although this may appear confusing, essentially they are offering the same service as for Gold OA journals but in a hybrid format. A study comparing citation rates for papers published with Hybrid OA, suggests that the $\sim$30% increased citations achieved is equivalent to the same citation increase obtained for making manuscripts available via Green OA (Piwowar et al., 2018). This should be an extra incentive to make an article available via an institutional repository, instead of paying a publisher for Hybrid OA.

A slight variation on hybrid OA is when you are a member of an academic society that allows its members to publish open access without extra payment. Students often get very discounted membership to an academic society which might make it very cheap to publish open access with them.

14.2.8   Platinum or Diamond OA

This is without doubt the best OA model, and the one that we should all strive for. In a platinum or diamond open access journal you do not have to pay any money but everything that is published is open access. In order to do this these journals are often subsidised by governmental or philanthropic agencies. Some university presses are also in the habit of publishing platinum or diamond OA when it meets with their stated mission. These journals are very rare but they do exist, and it is well worth looking for them.

Another great new model that is diamond OA is the concept of Overlay Journals. Although there aren't many overlay journals in the Biological Sciences at the time of writing.

14.2.9   Black OA

This refers to the placement of published material onto a pirate website such as Sci-Hub. Sci-Hub is considered by most governments to be illegal and may be blocked by your institution or country. However, many scientists all over the world depend on Sci-Hub in order to access literature and therefore conduct research. In addition, there are a number of other Black OA sites.

14.2.10 Grey OA

You can find grey OA repositories of published material on Academic Social Network sites in which you need membership to access such as ResearchGate (www.researchgate.net) and Academia.edu (www.academia.edu). The legality of such sites is regularly questioned (see Piwowar et al., 2018, for more details). There has been legal action with thousands of members being issues with take-down notices.

14.3   Supplementary information and data

Whichever route you decide to go for your manuscript, please do not place your data with the publisher. There are some examples where publishers choose to place both data and supplementary information deposited with them behind a paywall, even if the article is available Open Access. We also need to ask whether the publisher has the long-term vision to curate data, especially when the expense associated with this will rise over time as datasets accumulate behind their paywall. Elsewhere in this book you will find some suggestions about what to do with your data to make it available for all.

14.4   Unsure what you can legally do with a published paper?

If you don't know what level of copyright exists on something that you have published, then you can find an aggregated set of publisher policies at Sherpa Romeo (v2.sherpa.ac.uk/romeo/). This is a really nice database which provides a very simple summary by journal. You can also use this to check out a journal that you are thinking of publishing with. If you are still in doubt, then consult your librarian.

15

Submitting a paper to a journal for peer review

This chapter deals with the process of submitting a manuscript to a journal (Figure 15.1), and what to expect once this is done. It takes time to submit a paper using most existing editorial management software (see Hartley and Cabanac, 2017, for an overview). Detailed information is given on many of the parts, mentioned here, in later sections of the book. Be aware that although it does take a lot of effort to get a manuscript ready for submission (Hartley and Cabanac, 2017), once it is submitted, there is a lot more work taken on by a larger group of people who are (usually) not paid, and who are undertaking the work associated with your manuscript in addition to their 'day jobs'.

Most of the information required for submission is easy enough to provide, but they insist on having it entered in such an unfriendly way that it makes it all very painful. Believe it or not, they have improved over time. As this work is so tedious, it's worth reflecting why they need all of this information upfront before anyone even decides whether or not they want your paper. The reality is that all of this metadata (data associated with your manuscript) is really only of use if the manuscript is accepted. Otherwise, you are really just stuffing the database of the publisher full of information that they may (and likely will) use to spam you in the future. Some journals have actively reduced the amount of metadata that they require on initial submission (e.g. *eLife*), but this is not (yet) the norm. The only data that they must have on submission is your name and contact details, and the verification that you've adhered to the journal's ethical requirements (which you could do in a letter to the editor). Some of the rest will be of use to the editor when deciding who to allocate your submission to, but the vast majority of the metadata are only used if your article is accepted – and then they become vital.

Once accepted, metadata about your manuscript lies at the heart of the ability for CrossRef to link you, your co-authors and their ORCID accounts together with your manuscript using a DOI. All of this information is held in a header file of the published webpage so that Google Scholar can scrape it into their database. It's also used by all of your automated referencing software plugins. Having this data entered accurately means that the following processes will flow nicely. Doing a sloppy job will mean that those who rely on such services might well mis-cite your paper, get your name wrong, or one of lots of other potential

DOI: 10.1201/9781003220886-15

issues. Most of the major publishers now use this metadata to make up the author information (and addresses) on the front page of the typeset paper. Be aware that when they appear wrong on your proofs, it's likely because you (or the corresponding author) didn't enter the metadata correctly.

15.1 A typical submission workflow

The steps A to G (below) all refer back to letters in circles in Figure 15.1. Remember that most of the actions described below are also the subject of later sections in Parts II and III of this book.

A – formatting and submitting

- Targeting journals for submission: there are a lot of journals out there, and you need to make sure that you are submitting your manuscript to a journal in the right subject area (there is a detailed chapter on this subject). Remember to keep your ordered list of journals that you prepare so that you can refer back to this in the case of rejection.
- Prepare your manuscript according to the journal guidelines: this may require a lot of work especially if the journal requires full formatting on first submission. Some journals require additional items such as graphical abstracts, so make sure that you know what is needed before you start to submit. A checklist to run through before submission is available here, to which you should add any journal checklist from their instructions to authors. Circulate this final version among your co-authors. This is a good time to gather the needed meta-data for submission.
- Get all the files and metadata ready for submission. In addition to the manuscript, figures and tables, you'll (usually) need a cover letter, key-words, recommended (or opposed) reviewers, and addresses (with ORCID numbers) for all authors. All these items should already have met with the approval of your co-authors.
- For the purposes of this section, I am assuming that you are the corresponding author. This is something that you should learn to do. Being the corresponding author carries some extra duties as they are responsible for making sure that all the other authors are in agreement about the contents of the paper before submission. They are responsible for gathering all of the necessary information about each of the authors on the title page.
- Uploading your manuscript to the editorial management software requires time and preparation. Give yourself a good couple of hours for this process, and be aware that it can be frustrating. Friday afternoon might not be the best time. You may well need to refer back to your co-authors if you don't have their relevant information. As corresponding author, it is courteous

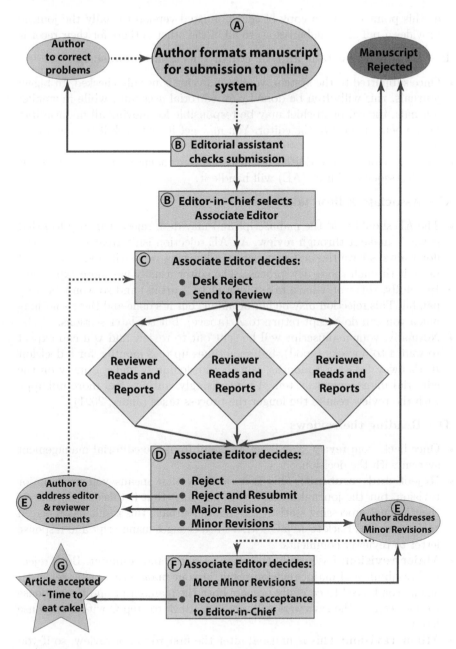

FIGURE 15.1: This schematic demonstrates the editorial workflow of a 'typical' journal. Ovals show actions by authors which have dotted lines, while rectangles show work done by the editorial team of the journal with solid lines. Referees are shown as diamonds. Letters in circles refer to the sections of the text (below). All arrows are potential places for delays.

at this point to send a copy of the submitted version (usually the journal provides a pdf of the submission) to all of the other authors for their records.

B – Editorial assistant and/or editor check the manuscript

- Once submitted to the system, your manuscript is usually checked. In bigger journals, this will often be done by an editorial assistant, while in smaller journals, the editor-in-chief may be responsible for moving all manuscripts. before being passed to the editor. You may get it sent back if the meta-data is wrong.
- Once the editor (often Editor-in-Chief) has your manuscript, they will decide which Associate Editor (AE) will handle it.

C – Associate Editor takes over

- The AE should read the manuscript and may desk reject it if they feel that it won't make it through review. An AE rejection isn't great news as AEs don't always have the best experience in knowing what will and what won't make it through the review process. The editor usually has more experience. Hopefully, this won't have taken long (1 to 2 weeks) and so won't be very painful. This rejection may be fair or unfair, but it's done and there's nothing much you can do except return to **A** (above), but see later sections.
- Normally, your manuscript will be sent out to review and you can expect to wait 4 to 6 weeks (good), but sometimes up to 3 months, for a decision. If it's away for over 3 months, you should definitely make a query on the editorial management system. Unsurprisingly, authors feel more unhappy with the review results the longer the process takes (Jiang, 2021).

D – Reading the reviews

- Once back from review, you'll get an email from the editorial management system with the decision.
- **Reject and resubmit:** This is a category that means you need major revision, but the journal doesn't want the time that it takes to do this on their journal processing statistics. In many journals, this result has replaced 'major revision'. Back to step C with a track changes manuscript and response letter to reviewer comments.
- **Major revision:** Essentially the same as reject and resubmit. Both reject and resubmit and major revision result in your manuscript being reviewed again. You'll need to carefully prepare both the manuscript and the response to reviewers as the reviewers will see both. Back to step C with a response letter.
- **Minor revision:** This is unusual after the first round of review, so if you get this decision first time it's something to celebrate. You may have already done one (or more) rounds of Major revision before you get here. After addressing the Minor revisions, your manuscript should now only be assessed by the AE, so you should address your responses to them.

- **Accept without further revision:** This is practically unheard of on first submission. Your manuscript may have already undergone some peer review (maybe as a preprint or at another journal), or in previous rounds of review. This decision is likely a recommendation from the AE to the Editor-in-Chief.

E – Revising and resubmitting your manuscript

- If you are resubmitting, aim to prioritise this to get it done in 2 to 3 weeks if possible.
- The reason is that the same reviewers are likely to be willing to look at your manuscript again within a month, and will remember all the points that they made. Similarly, the AE will remember all of the issues that they had. It's hard to stress how valuable this is, as keeping it all fresh will result in a swift response.
- If you don't or can't manage to get your responses back quickly, you might expect a rocky ride through the review process when you go back for the second round. The reviewers you had before might not be available, but the AE will be obliged to have at least 2 reviews again. This means that you may get new reviews. New reviewers are likely to throw up new issues, and could result in your manuscript getting rejected at this stage, or that you'll have another Major revision decision, sending you back to step C with a track changes manuscript and response letter to reviewer comments. This drags the whole process on for much longer and reviewers and AEs are likely to look less favourably at your manuscript.
- A better result is when there are only Minor revisions. In this case the manuscript is simply bouncing between you and the AE and even if this happens more than once, it's fine as long as you can keep the response time reasonable (within a couple of weeks).
- In either case, your rebuttal letter will be a very important part of your resubmission, and this will be covered in a later section.

F – Associate Editor recommends to Editor-in-Chief

- When the AE is happy with all of your Minor Revisions, they will make a recommendation to the Editor-in-Chief. The Editor-in-Chief may have some extra revisions that they would like to see, but these will likely be minor.
- It is unlikely that the Editor-in-Chief would disagree with the acceptance of any paper that an AE has signed off on.
- It is worth bearing in mind that the Editor-in-Chief does have the final say on whether or not your manuscript can be accepted to the journal.

G – Acceptance

- Hopefully your manuscript will now be accepted, and you are entering the last stages of the process. Your accepted manuscript should be sent to the publishers for copy editing and typesetting, and you can get the proofs back very quickly (for some publishers). Most demand that the proofs are returned very quickly (often within 48 hours), and you should try to prioritise this if you can. If you can, please also send the proof to the co-authors. The more eyes the better at this stage for spotting errors. Don't expect to be able to change a lot in the proof process, it's really just for catching errors. Carefully check all figures, tables and legends. It's not unknown that typesetters cause problems when they make proofs (tables can be disasters). A detailed section is provided in Part III on what to do once your manuscript is accepted.

- If you (or a co-author) spot a fundamental error with your data or analyses at this point (or any of the other steps above), you should discuss it with all co-authors and decide what to do. It's better to withdraw the manuscript now than to have to retract it later (see part IV).

Rejected

- If your manuscript is Rejected, take the comments of the reviewers on board. Think about it for a couple of days, and then set about revising the manuscript. However unfair you think the reviewers have been, there should be some important messages for you to consider carefully and discuss among the co-authors before going back to step A with the next journal on your list. More information to reflect on regarding a rejection is provided in a later section.

15.1.1   Remember that peer review is conducted by humans

The peer review process is not ideal, but it is worth remembering that it's there to help improve your manuscript. The most prominent problems involve the time that the editorial team take to find reviewers and have them agree to complete reviews in a timely manner. In Figure 15.1, only 4 of the arrows are in the control of the authors, while at least 16 are within the editorial management process. Each one could be the source of your manuscript getting stuck. Throughout the process, you should be able to track the progress of your manuscript using the editorial management software online. More information on delays in the handling of manuscripts is provided in a later section.

16

Expectations of peer review?

Once your manuscript is submitted and has passed the initial rounds of checks (A to C in Figure 15.1), you can expect that you will receive a written review of your manuscript. Sometimes, you may also receive an annotated manuscript back, but you can interpret this in your own way – most likely as minor comments.

It is widely acknowledged that peer reviews are likely to be biased in some way, and so you should expect this of every review that you get. Try to look over these biases and aim to receive the wisdom that they likely also contain.

16.1 What are peer reviewers asked to do?

The peer review report consists of three major parts: the review, confidential comments to the editor, and the reviewer's opinion of what decision should be made. You will only have access to the first of these three. Understanding peer review is greatly aided by conducting peer review, which is covered by a section in Part IV. Reading about how to conduct peer review may help with your interpretation of the reviews that you receive.

16.1.1 The review

Peer reviewers should sum up the manuscripts in their own words to demonstrate that they have understood the contents. This is important because being able to summarise what you have read demonstrates the reviewer's comprehension. If the reviewer gets this summary wrong, then it is either a flag to the editor that they lacked the necessary comprehension to make their review meaningful. Or, because there are two sides to comprehension, a flag to the authors that they failed to write their manuscript in a way that made it easy for the reader to comprehend.

DOI: 10.1201/9781003220886-16

The reviewer should then provide a general critique including positive and any negative aspects of the manuscript. They should provide detailed information on exactly how the manuscript should be improved, including any significant literature that might be missing from the manuscript. Lastly, they can provide a list of minor comments along the length of the manuscript that require further attention from the authors. When I undertake this last part, I tend to do it with page and line numbers (which is one reason why submitting a manuscript with line numbers is so important). If the minor comments get too numerous, then I tend to stick with major comments.

16.1.2   Reviewer's confidential comments to the editor

The reviewers are provided with a box where they can write to the editor without text being seen by the authors. It is worth bearing in mind that the editor can act on these (unseen) comments. I'm not a big fan of confidential comments but sometimes they are warranted. Many reviewers avoid making comments in these boxes, in accordance with trends for transparency.

16.1.3   Reviewer's opinion and the editorial decision

In many journals, the reviewers are directly asked whether the manuscript should be rejected or resubmitted (major or minor revisions). This opinion is given in a set of 'radio buttons' in the editorial management software. Depending on the journal, a number of additional qualitative questions are asked of reviewers that may be pivotal to the progress of a manuscript. These questions are set by the gatekeepers for the journal in question, and may ask whether the manuscript is worthy of publication in that journal, in the top 5% of important findings, or similar. Bornmann and Marx (2012) found that some journals require that all reviewers respond with a positive criterion on these questions, or the manuscript will not be considered further. They term this the 'Anna Karenina Principle' (AKP) of peer review because it requires 'positive selection' on all criteria, whereas previously papers were selected by meeting minimum standards; 'negative selection', which is now the overriding principle for 'no Impact Factor' journals.

Unless you know someone who can tell you the editorial practice of the journal you submitted to, you will not know whether or not your manuscript has been judged on the answers to these questions. However, if you receive all positive reviews and a rejection, it may well be that one or more of the positive reviewers did not select a criterion high enough on one of these questions. Personally, I don't think that reviewers should be asked these subjective questions, as this potentially trivialises decision making for gatekeepers. Editors must read the manuscript and all reviewer comments in order to reach decisions. Certainly, all journals need to provide transparent criteria for selection of manuscripts, without which the black box nature via AKP workings of peer review will only perpetuate.

16.2   What do good reviews look like?

Good reviews are those where authors improve their manuscript. It may be that the good review doesn't immediately show the way on the first reading (although clearly the best ones should), but it may be that the authors require some work rethinking their manuscript before they understand the comments of a reviewer. I would say that usually on first reading, even a good review might not sound that good.

16.2.1   The myth of the 'shit sandwich'

The shit sandwich is a review where the beginning and end are generally positive, while the very critical appraisal happens in the middle. Although the shit sandwich might be seen as a way for a reviewer to sugar coat their negative message, an analysis of *PLOS ONE* reviews by Eve et al. (2021) suggests that some of the best reviews (think Minor Revisions) actually have this format. Here the reviewer will be positive in the outset and the summing up, but then in the middle have a set of issues that need correcting. Hence, they found that the shit in the shit sandwich wasn't that bad. In the same analysis, Eve et al. (2021) found that truly bad (i.e. Reject) reviews could be bad at any point in their length.

16.3   What are reviewers not asked to do?

In their analysis of *PLOS ONE* reviews, Eve et al. (2021) found that reviewers are good at ignoring the directions that are provided to them by the journal. It is therefore necessary to be aware of what reviewers are not asked to do, because sometimes they do it anyway!

Peer review is not a trial by committee. Those of you who have experienced manuscripts being critiqued at a journal club will know that there are very few published papers that leave a journal club without having many negative, critical comments. Instead peer review is conducted by an individual, on their own and with their own personal limitations. Peer reviewers are forbidden from sharing the contents of a manuscript with others, without express permission from the editor.

Reviewers are not required to correct English grammar. It's not the job of a reviewer to correct any faulty grammar on a manuscript. Similarly it is not up to the reviewer to correct stylistic aspects of the manuscript. However, as English is such a subjective language, it is important that ambiguity is removed, and grammatical aspects can be important for this.

I have noted that some reviewers have become quite obsessive about things like the Oxford comma – insisting that the Oxford comma should be inserted at every possible juncture. Eve et al. (2021) call these reviewers 'peer copyeditors'. They are likely to comment on your split infinitives and may be pedants for all grammatical concerns.

I would say that it is up to you as an author to decide whether the suggestions from these 'peer copyeditors' are warranted. At the same time, the comments from these same people might drastically improve the readability of your manuscript.

Reviewers should not instruct authors to cite their papers. Sadly, this is something that a lot of peer reviewers do, and are part of a suite of not-so-legitimate ways in which people manipulate citations. The reviewers' own work can be cited, but only when relevant, and the authors should be able to choose whether or not they want to make any additional citations.

Reviewers and gatekeepers should not instruct authors to cite other papers from the journal. This also happens, see section on Impact Factor, often at the request of the editor. It is part of IF manipulation, and you should not act on this.

Peer review should always be an objective critique of a manuscript. It's not really the place of the reviewer to express their opinion or their beliefs about a particular study that they are reviewing. Watch out for statements that begin with 'I believe. . . ' or 'In my opinion. . . '.

Reviewers should stick to the evidence that they're provided with. If they are not provided with sufficient evidence then they should draw attention to the lack of information rather than extrapolate to what they believe might be the case.

Authors should be provided the benefit of the doubt and opportunity to respond to such criticisms especially when information is missing. It's unfair for reviewers to act as judge and jury. This is the job of the editor.

Reviewers should not assess aspects of the manuscript beyond their competence. Some manuscripts are cross-cutting across several subjects or may contain analyses outside it with the experience of a reviewer. In these cases reviewers should not attempt to review areas that are beyond their competence. Instead they should bring these aspects to the attention of the editor when they are submitting their review.

Reviewers should not ignore what is good. It is often thought that peer review provides only negative criticism (see Eve et al., 2021). This should not be the case as peer reviewers should also be able to accentuate the positive aspects of manuscripts that they read. Even if a manuscript is not considered acceptable, the positive attributes should be bought the attention of the editors as well as those that are negative.

It is important for authors to understand what aspects of their manuscript are good. This kind of feedback from peer review will likely influence future versions of this manuscript as well as future studies from these research groups.

17

Receiving the editor's decision

Peer review is the basis of guarding and maintaining quality in science. If you've just got a decision from a journal, you'll need to respond to the comments. This to and fro between authors and reviewers usually doesn't exceed two rounds. As you approach the comments, there are several points that it's worth bearing in mind:

- The task of the reviewer is to help improve your manuscript for the scientific record and for the reader
- The reviewers and editors have given their time freely to help you and your work
- It's easy to misinterpret what reviewers and editors say, and you need to take the time and space to respond appropriately

If you already know what it's like to receive reviewer comments, but struggle to understand why reviewers say what they do, then it's time for you to start reviewing papers. You can ask your mentor to mention you as a potential reviewer (especially if they are going to decline because they are too busy). But probably the best way to get started is to participate with your lab or journal club in the review of a preprint (see Part II). This has the advantage that you are not the sole reviewer, but will be in a group. Your group will get credit for their review (via a DOI). You will get to discuss the finer points of reviewing with your team. Especially, you will likely hear remarks that might come across as insulting or unprofessional and it'll give you a chance to challenge these at source, and so positively influence others.

17.1 What to expect in your decision letter

When you finally receive it, the email will contain some stock text about the overall decision, some information about how to resubmit your revised version (if you have this as an option), and a time-frame. After the editor has signed off, you will find comments first from the Associate Editor (AE) who handled the review, and then from (typically) two reviewers, but sometimes three (or even more). It would be a good idea to add the deadline to your calender,

DOI: 10.1201/9781003220886-17

especially if you feel that you won't be able to respond immediately. You can always ask for an extention if you are likely to go over the allotted time.

17.1.1   The desk rejection

A desk rejection is when your manuscript is assessed by a subject editor (it could be the editor-in-chief, an associate editor or any rank in between), and they decide (based on your title, abstract, cover letter, or a quick look at the content), that the manuscript is: not in the right subject area, insufficiently novel (too many similar papers), or unlikely to make it through peer review (not scientifically robust). The editor in question should explain how your manuscript failed to meet the specified editorial requirements for undergoing peer review in their journal (Teixeira da Silva et al., 2018). In my experience, this is rarely the case. Instead, it appears as if these editors are making a quick confirmation bias decisions based on whether or not they consider the submission will receive sufficient interest in order to match their Impact Factor (or even inflate it). Moreover, it has been suggested that these decisions by editors are on the whole poor, with 66% of submissions being accepted in an equivalent journal without changes (Farji-Brener and Kitzberger, 2014). The editors responded that their desk rejections are far more nuanced, and that equivalent journals don't necessarily have the same scope (Schimel et al., 2014). You should have already checked the scope of the journal prior to submission. The reality is that many journals have far too many submissions than they can handle, and so there is a need for an initial triage. In general, desk rejections work well for all concerned when authors know why they have received this decision. For this, there need to be specific guidelines that are followed consistently by the whole editorial team (Teixeira da Silva et al., 2018).

On the positive side, a desk rejection is fast (otherwise, it's unfair) and there should be plenty more journals on your list. It is possible to appeal, but you will already have had an editorial decision against your manuscript, hence you will be fighting an uphill battle from the start. In terms of your time and effort, you'd probably be better off accepting this rejection and moving on.

17.1.2   Take a rejection seriously

Rejections are harsh, but totally normal (Cassey and Blackburn, 2004; Day, 2011). Everyone gets rejections, including the top scientists in their fields (Cassey and Blackburn, 2003). As a result, you will feel disheartened, frustrated and even angry (Pannell, 2002), and this is normal too. Don't take it personally, and you'll find that the more you share the times you fail, the more you'll find that others share the experience (Crew, 2019). You will need to pick yourself up, and take your manuscript back and try again. The results of a survey among top ecologists suggests that scientists need to develop a thick skin when it comes to rejection (Cassey and Blackburn, 2003). Learn as many lessons as you can from your rejection and quickly move on. Certainly, never dwell on a rejection and feel that this is anything more than a minor setback. Receiving a rejection is not an indication of professional inadequacy, also known as imposter syndrome (Woolston, 2016). All of us have been rejected, and continue to deal with rejections throughout our careers.

The most important point to discern as quickly as possible is whether or not your manuscript is not fundamentally flawed. If you receive a rejection because your study is flawed then take the time to learn the lesson. This will be a hard lesson to accept because it speaks about your experimental design, and whether or not you can really answer the questions that you set out to when forming your hypothesis.

Do not start Hypothesising After Results are Known (HARKing). If you have made mistakes in your experimental design, then your data might be useful for a post-hoc manuscript. There is no shame in producing a descriptive note of this kind. Many researchers appear to automatically send a flawed manuscript to another journal to see how it will do there. These manuscripts are very plentiful and take up the time of a great many people (in specialist areas you see them doing the rounds of different journals). I would urge you to learn from mistakes, and not to burden others with them. Many editors try to give good advice when making rejections, and you should take the time needed to absorb this. If you believe their assessment to be wrong, and it may be, then seek out some honest sounding boards for your manuscript, such as a mentor or another colleague or post-doc.

Sometimes, you will receive a Reject decision, and the editors' comments will allude to the work not being sufficiently novel, or not sufficiently advancing the field. In other words, whatever it was that they were looking for, your manuscript didn't have it. Tacked onto the end of their email may be the offer to submit to another journal in the same stable, the so-called 'portable peer review'. Typically, these are Open Access No Impact Factor journals where you have to pay an, often hefty, article processing charge to get published. This is rarely a good idea. The standings of these journals are (typically) not great, and you'd probably be better off going back to your original submission list and selecting the next journal there. Having said this, if the journal offers to move your submission with or without the peer reviews, at least you know that your manuscript is not fundamentally flawed. This kind of rejection is simply an example of publication bias, and it is time for you to move on from this journal to another on your submission list.

17.1.3   Time taken to receive your decision

Usually, you will receive a decision letter (email) after ~60 days. This depends on the journal, editors and reviewers, but it's worth signing into the editorial management system and looking at the status of your manuscript. If after 60 days the status hasn't changed and you've heard nothing, then contact the editorial team (with the email address given in the editorial management system). Time to first decision in the Life Sciences was found to average 11 weeks and 25% of decisions are received within a month (Huisman and Smits, 2017). That might sound oh so slow, but this is relatively quick when compared to the 18 week average first response in economics.

It is worth bearing in mind that authors generally feel more unhappy with the reviewer comments they receive the longer they have to wait (Jiang, 2021), while fast turn around times produce more content authors even in the face of rejections (Huisman and Smits, 2017). Clearly, the difference is in the resentment of time wasted, especially for a desk rejection, or even for poor or feeble reviewer input with a rejection. If you feel particularly unhappy about long waiting times, then you could consider releasing your manuscript as a preprint. Otherwise, there's little that you can do, and it can simply be bad luck when you have to wait a long time for a review. Different journals have different mean times to first decision, and some (often those with faster times) advertise this and so this may influence your decision about where to take your manuscript next.

In my experience, every manuscript is different and it's very hard as an editor to determine how long it will take to find reviewers, or how long those reviewers will take to produce their reviews. Just because reviewers accept to undertake reviews, does not mean that they will do them timeously, or even at all. After a failure to review on time, a good editor will follow up to seek out other potential reviewers. But there are other reasons why decisions may take time.

In the case that the editor found no reviewers after looking for some weeks, one option is for them to make a 'desk reject' and encourage resubmission. In the rejection, they may point out a number of potentially minor faults. For the editor, it takes the heat off of their desk. They may not be allocated the new manuscript after resubmission. For the authors, it's just frustrating. If you suspect this has happened then consider another journal (with a clear editorial stance on peer review), or provide more potential reviewers.

It is worth remembering that certain times of the year are likely to take longer than others for peer review. Editors find it more difficult to find reviewers in the summer months when many biologists are in the field or on holiday (remember that summer occurs at different times in northern and southern hemispheres). The start of the academic year is also a particularly busy time for most academics (editors and reviewers), and you might expect to wait longer (although academic years start at different times in different countries).

In general, academics are busy and finding reviewers is difficult (Perry et al., 2012).

The delay from the end of data collection to being published can take between 0.5 and 3.5 years, depending on the subdiscipline of Biological Sciences that you are working in (Christie et al., 2021). This includes the initial write-up and submission time, together with any initial rejections from other journals and multiple rounds of reviews. This adds to many other arguments for using preprint servers to make your work publicly available as soon as it is completed (Christie et al., 2021).

17.2 What to do when you receive your reviewer comments

Your reviewer comments will arrive in an email when you are busy doing something else. If you have time to read them the same day, then my suggestion is that you read without trying anything further. Remember to forward them to your co-authors as soon as possible. Simply read the comments and then close the email and mark it for further attention the next day. Your writing is very personal to you, and you might be surprised at just how hurtful it can feel to have someone critique your writing (and your experiment) without holding back. If you've not experienced this before, then prepare yourself. No matter how much effort you put into your text, sending it out for peer review is a really high bar. Make an appointment with your co-authors so that you can discuss the comments together. Whether good, bad, or bizarre, it is best to set aside some time to read through the comments carefully, so that you can respond.

17.3 Responding to reviewers' comments with a rebuttal

The reviewers are usually given two boxes to write comments in. One pertains to the comments that you receive in your letter, and the second is for the confidential comments to the Associate Editor (AE). Remember that the AE is acting on both of these sets of comments, and so the decision may reflect something that is said in confidence. This is not really in the spirit of transparency for peer review. The best peer review systems are open and online.

Once you've found the time in your week, sooner is better than later, sit and read the comments again. Normally, they will sound much better, and less harsh, on the second read (if not, try third or fourth). They should seem far more approachable than when you first read them. Most reviews will have a set of major (when applicable) and minor comments that you need to address from each of them. Try sketching a few responses down to the major revision comments before your meeting with your co-authors. The easiest way to do this is to copy all of the comments from the email (together with those of the editor), and paste them all into a fresh document. Use a different colour text or a clear set of symbols (e.g. »») to indicate which text is your response and which is the reviewers' or editors'. Or number each comment and reply. If it isn't clear enough, then the editor may well get confused about what is the comment and what is the rebuttal. One of the best ways I've seen of doing this was to make a table with all the comments in one column (each on a separate row), and the author responses in a new column.

Sketch out your responses to the major comments, and use a tick if you are happy with making the suggested minor comments. If there are comments that you don't know how to handle, simply leave them with a question mark. By making this start before you meet with your co-authors, you will have an idea of what is likely to be difficult to tackle in the revision. Even if you've received a rejection with reviewers' comments, it's well worth having this same meeting with your co-authors so that you can decide together what to do next. Skipping on comments from reviewers during a rejection appears to be very common (Crijns et al., 2021), but is a very uncollegial way of moving forward. I have personally reviewed manuscripts that were rejected, only to see them again as a reviewer in another journal with all of the same errors.

Make a plan of how to handle all of the comments, or where to go, what to read or who to talk to (perhaps another co-author), to sort out those you don't know. Decide whether you need to send out the journal decision to co-authors now, or wait until you have your rebuttal ready to circulate. For me this decision is largely based on how much time the revision is likely to take: if it's quick, rather send the revision and rebuttal together with the decision.

Next, when you sit down to write the rebuttal and revise the document, you need to make sure that you have pressed 'track changes' on the submitted version of the manuscript. I find it easiest to have both the rebuttal letter and the revised manuscript open side by side on the screen. As you revise the manuscript in response to the comment, make a note to mark that it's done in the rebuttal letter. Mark any comments that you don't do. Your revision is written as a rebuttal to the editor. While you don't write your comments back to the reviewer, it is worth bearing in mind that the reviewer is likely to read them.

Three watchwords should be your guides for your response to the reviewers:

professional – polite – precise

In addition to these, make the entire process easier for everyone by:

- Making a note of the line number where the revision is made (note that these can shift around in the revision)
- If you have reworded the text, do copy and paste that rewording into the rebuttal using quotes and corresponding line numbers
- Simply use a word like 'done' to indicate changes on Minor comments
- Do be polite with your responses, you don't get any extra points for wordy thankfulness or praise. Keep it succinct and to the point
- Signal when you agree with the comment and that you have made a change to the text

Reviewers sometimes use a chatty style, and it may appear to you that they are asking you a question. For example, they might ask you exactly how accurate a piece of equipment you used to measure your organism. Intuitively, it seems like the right thing to do is to simply answer them in the rebuttal. But they expect you to make a change to the manuscript, and not simply to give them an answer in the rebuttal. Otherwise, it would have been pointless in making the comment.

Do bear in mind that your reviewer is a human, and was likely operating under less than ideal conditions when reading your manuscript. They could have been getting constant interruptions. They could have been reading it after having read another three manuscripts. They could suffer from insomnia and read it in the middle of the night with no sleep for a week. Give the reviewer the benefit of the doubt. Do remember to thank your reviewers and editors in your acknowledgements. They've been working and doing the best for your manuscript without any thanks other than what you will give them. So give them a boost and help make their day that much brighter.

17.3.1 What if you don't agree with a reviewer?

Most of the time, reviewer comments are sensible, helpful and genuine attempts at improving the quality of your contribution. If you don't agree with particular points, try skipping them and moving ahead with the easy points or those that you do agree with. Discuss any points that you don't agree with your co-authors. Try to get another perspective on the comment. Do your best to try to see the comment from the reviewers standpoint.

For example, a reviewer might ask for details on a point in the methods, but they are mentioned in another section of the methods. This is a cue for you to add a flag to that point in the manuscript. For example, write: 'see section 2.2.3 for an explanation of how this was done'.

If a reviewer has made a comment that says that they don't understand something, this means that you need to make a change in your text so that the text is easier to understand. If they don't understand, then it could be that more people don't understand and you want your text to be understood by all people that are reading it, so make a change.

If you and your co-authors don't agree with the reviewer, then make it clear what exactly you don't agree with. Again, try to see it from the reviewer's perspective and write a courteous and clear explanation of why they might have misunderstood or misinterpreted what was written. Back up your comments with citations, even if these aren't cited in the paper. Provide full references for any citations you give. The more thorough your explanation of both sides of the disagreement, the more likely the editor will side with your perspective on the point that you don't agree with. You may find that you want to include some of this text in the manuscript, or that you offer to provide it in the Supplementary Information (if there's a word limit on the manuscript).

Remember that the reviewer is likely to read exactly what you write in your rebuttal. Your job is to professionally explain why you don't agree. Forget any of the emotions that you might believe to be there. Revert back to professionalism, because you are a professional.

17.3.2   When reviewers ask for additional analyses or experiments

It is not unusual for reviewers to suggest additional or different analyses, or even experiments. It will be important for you, as author, to differentiate between requests that are reasonable and stay within the original bounds of your stated hypothesis, and those that do not. Because there are so many ways in which to analyse data, it is not unusual for a reviewer to suggest you use their preferred method over the one that you submitted. Such suggestions are made with good intentions, and unless there are clear reasons for not undertaking these analyses (such as you have already preregistered your study or they are inappropriate), you should attempt the analyses and then make a call on whether or not they improve your work. Even if you decide not to include the results, you can present them to the reviewer/editor in your rebuttal, together with your reasoning for not including them.

It is important to be aware of P-hacking even in your rebuttal. Improving your work through peer review should not result in changing the focus of your work, or even including a co-variate that you did not plan to use. Many authors feel pushed into conducting extra analyses for fear of having their manuscript rejected (Hopewell et al., 2018). Although it's impossible to determine every potential scenario here, if your work was well prepared and conceived, you should not need to conduct extra experiments and there should be journal policy to prevent this.

Exceptions might include when journals ask for independent experimentation to determine a mechanism detected (or speculated on) in the manuscript. Including multiple lines of evidence is likely to have your article accepted with higher impact. You may or may not have the option of doing this kind of extra work, and may therefore need to settle for another journal. In all cases, discussions with your co-authors should help you decide on the best course of action.

17.3.3 When reviewers don't agree

Normally, you will have two reviews (possibly three depending on the journal policy) and comments from the AE. The AE acts as a judge given the opinions of the reviewers, and so if the reviewers disagree, the AE should suggest the correct direction for you to take. Sometimes this means that the AE will consult a third reviewer (and occasionally even more reviewers). This is one of the many reasons why it is important for editors to read your work. If the AE gives you no direction (as is increasingly the case) then make this decision with your co-authors and indicate to the AE the conflict between the reviewers and the reason why you've chosen the direction you have.

17.3.4 More than two rounds of peer review

You should not expect to have more than two rounds of peer review for most articles, but there are instances when this could happen. There are plenty of reasons why your manuscript might go into extra rounds of peer review, chief among these is the acquisition of new reviewers' after others are unavailable. However, the AE should be doing everything that they can to avoid this. In cases where it happens, you should be receiving helpful and specific comments from your AE. In the instance that you are making all possible changes to reviewer comments, but not receiving a clear and directed decision from your AE after three rounds of review, you can reasonably appeal to the Editor-in-Chief.

Note that on occasion it is the authors that are refusing to implement changes in the manuscript demanded by reviewers and editors. In this case, you should expect that your manuscript will be rejected. The most common problem that I see is that editors fail to state exactly what they want. Then the authors and reviewers end up in unnecessary rounds of reviews.

17.3.5   Is your reviewer being unprofessional?

Reviewers' comments can come across as harsh, upsetting, rude and even arrogant. While it isn't ok for reviewers to be rude, it does sometimes happen (see Part IV). If you really feel that a reviewer is being unprofessional, it is worth flagging this with the editor. I've never had to do this myself, but I am aware that there is some unprofessional behaviour out there (I've seen it on ShitMyReviewersSay: shitmyreviewerssay.tumblr.com). Discuss it with your co-authors, but here are two potential options:

- If it's just one or two comments, then simply indicate to the editor that you don't feel that you know how to respond. Ask the reviewer to try again, or ask the editor to interpret the comment for you.
- If it is every comment from one reviewer, write an email to the handling editor and ask for their guidance. You should find their email address in the journal submission site. They will flag it with the editor and come back with a solution for you.

17.3.6   Appealing against a decision that you think is unfair

From time to time, a decision comes from an editor that is clearly unfair. I've had a few. As I've mentioned before, scientists are humans and humans do have biases that manifest into their professional lives. This is the reason for double-blind review. Scientists in STEM are predominantly white and male, and express the views of this minority but powerful group. Their prejudices are evident in some decisions, and it is important to push back against this when you feel that this is the reason for a decision.

Most (good) journals will have an appeals process and you should look this up and see what's involved. While doing this, it is worth reviewing the journal's policy on how they handle manuscripts; again, good journals should have a clear policy. Of all the rejections and poor decisions I've had on my manuscripts over the years, I've only felt that decisions were unfair and worth appealing two or three times.

Normally, an appeal is made to the editor in chief. Be very clear about why you are appealing and what in the decision does not tally with the journal's own policy. Remain professional and detached from the decision itself and instead appeal on how the journal's own policy was not followed. For example, a journal may have a policy that the editor will sum up all of the reviewers' comments and use this as the basis for their decision. If the editor seems to have sided with one reviewer while not considering others, this can be the basis of an appeal.

Any appeal should be agreed with your co-authors before sending it.

18

Why should an editor read your submission?

There is a worrying increase in poor editorial decision making because editors are not reading submissions. In their survey of Associate Editors, Poulson-Ellestad et al. (2020) advised Early Career Researchers not to take on the position of Associate Editor unless they know that they have enough time in their jobs. This is an assessment with which I agree. You must be prepared to carve out dedicated time in which you can concentrate several times a week, or nearly every day for the Editor-in-Chief.

When a manuscript is submitted to a journal, the submission goes to either the editor-in-chief or a handling editor based on the key words or journal section implied during submission (see Part II). In some journals (like *PeerJ*) the submissions are offered up to a whole group of editors who can take their pick. It seems that the next thing that happens is that the manuscript is sent out for peer review. But stop. That's not correct and it's really not a good way to proceed. Before sending it out, the designated handling editor needs to read the submission.

18.1 Why is reading so important?

The title and abstract really don't allow a handling editor to decide whether or not a manuscript should go out to review. There are a lot of manuscripts out there that should not have been submitted, because their authors do not have sufficient judgement of their own or because they believe that there is a reason to just 'chance it' (especially if the manuscript has been rejected by somewhere else already). It is very important that handling editors read the submission, because without that they are moving editorial responsibility from themselves to the peer reviewers.

Some years ago, I co-authored a series of articles (Perry et al., 2012) that were published across many journals about how peer review was becoming very difficult for editors because so few colleagues accept to do reviews. This was a problem then, and it's a problem that has grown in time. I've recently sent out manuscripts to more than 15 people before getting two reviewers accept the invitation. That peers are not prepared to review, or in many cases even to respond to the request, is very poor. However, more recently I'm experiencing a sharp increase in manuscripts to review that should never have been sent out.

My time is precious, and it's becoming quite expensive for my employers. I am happy to conduct peer review because it is an important part of the scientific publishing process, and I expect others to review my own work. However, I expect that any manuscript that I receive is worthy of my attention and time. If the handling editor has not read it, they cannot decide this and I really wonder what makes them think that they can send it to me (and presumably others) to read while they don't feel that they have time to do it themselves. Moreover, this appears to be a trend among younger, less experienced, editors (often Associate Editors) that have not received any guidance in what their job as editor is, or how to do it.

18.2   Editors must be prepared to read

I must admit that I've done it. I've sent out manuscripts to be reviewed even when I didn't have the time to properly read the article myself. A superficial skim suggested that it seemed fine. Not good. It's embarrassing to have sent out manuscripts that should be rejected without peer review. In the case I'm thinking of, once I'd found time to read through the manuscript later on that day, I realised how bad it was and immediately wrote to those I'd asked to do the reviews and asked them not to. The article was rejected. It is important that this burden is taken on by the editor than burden two or three times as many other reviewers to make the same call.

Sometimes, it's not clear whether or not a manuscript will pass muster. Articles can stand or fall on good or bad single judgements of the authors. But misjudgements aren't always obvious to editors. That's why peer review is important, and that's why it's hugely important for editors to send manuscripts to appropriate reviewers who have some expertise in a subject.

Science is built on the work that others have done before, but basing your work on what someone else has written will mean that you have a good understanding of what they have done and how they have done it. Assumptions have to be made to get anything done, and it's a good exercise to sit down with a published paper (or even a manuscript of a colleague or your own) and read through listing all the assumptions that are made. Physicists might have a very long list if they read a biologist's manuscript, but with some practice you learn to see the assumptions that the authors have made when designing their experiment, or going out to the field to conduct their study. An incorrect assumption could lead to the entire manuscript losing its value.

18.3 I've been on the other end too

I've submitted manuscripts to journals where the editor clearly never read the manuscript. Editors who have made a decision without any guidance of their own gives this away. If your decision comes as a single sentence that asks you to revise according to the reviewers' comments, then you can be reasonably sure that your editor hasn't read the manuscript (and possibly not even the reviews).

It's not surprising that the editors have little to nothing to say; without reading the manuscript, the reviewer comments aren't really very helpful. Without reading, the editor has no idea whether the reviewer is biased. As an editor, you simply have to read. And if you don't have time to read, you shouldn't be an editor.

18.4 There is worse that goes on in economics

If the above makes some editors in Biological Sciences look bad, then I apologise. Being an editor for a journal is a pretty thankless task and there is no financial gain when doing an editorial stint. However, if you're going to do it, then you must do it well. The half measures that I describe above are simply not good enough. But biological journals are a huge cut above those in economics. I've always had my doubts about economics as a subject. Rather like theology, it's based on a fanciful construct that puts its own practitioners in positions of power when we'd do just as well to flip a coin.

In May 2018, I was pursued for some weeks by the *International Journal of Finance and Economics* to conduct a review of an article submitted there. Even though I raised the flag that I was not an appropriate reviewer, the editorial assistant (not the editor) still wanted me to conduct the review. Apparently, 'the system recommended me' and this was enough for me to be selected. It appears that the problem of non-expert reviewers is on the increase. Consider this blog post by Ivan Oransky (2021), one of the authors of Retraction Watch who was invited to review papers on COVID-19! Essentially, this is the result of editorial management systems 'auto-suggesting' reviewers, and editors not doing their due diligence to determine whether any of these reviewers is worthy of conducting peer review on that submission.

Clearly, selection of reviewers must be done by the handling editor, and those people must be chosen based on their expertise (not lack of it). While editorial management systems might help editors, they can't replace diligence on behalf of those who are responsible for the upholding integrity of the peer review system.

18.5   Summing up on editorial blunders

The way to get round making the kind of editorial blunders I describe above is simply for editors to read their manuscripts. The guidance of how to read a manuscript should be explained to editors when they take up the position. There is plenty of information out there on the internet, but the journal's editorial policy should be understood by all of the editors (and preferably open to authors and reviewers too), and that should include reading manuscripts before sending them out for peer review.

Part III

After your paper is accepted

19

Now that your manuscript has been accepted

This part of the book gives you information on some actions that you might want to do after your paper is accepted for publication. Much of this section is concerned with publicising the results and content beyond academia and for non-academic audiences. Even if you feel that there would be no interest beyond your academic niche, it would still be worth making some effort to publicise and popularise your study.

19.1 The Version of Record

An important concept to understand in the publication of your article is the Version of Record (VoR). This is the final typeset version of your article that is published.

In this millennium, the VoR had changed from a hard copy, that was printed and bound into an issue of a journal, into a pdf that appears at a journal website online. In addition, the VoR no longer has to belong to a volume or an issue, and is usually the first version available online (Haustein et al., 2015). The VoR can appear online long before it appears in an issue or volume (i.e. without page numbers), but still be the VoR.

If the publisher is a CrossRef (www.crossref.org) member (most are), they will register the content and assign it a Digital Object Identifier (DOI).

19.1.1 What does having a VoR mean?

- This means that if you wanted to make any changes to this first printed version (the VoR), you'd need to publish a separate corrigendum
- The date of the VoR has an impact on primacy
- In taxonomy, for example, if there are two descriptions of a species, the earliest one counts as the valid one

DOI: 10.1201/9781003220886-19

20

Once your paper is accepted

The day your paper is accepted, tell your co-authors. If they are in the same physical location as you then buy a cake, and celebrate with them at tea time. If cake isn't your thing, then find another appropriate treat for you and your co-authors. It's a great achievement and something you should share together. If you aren't in the same location then make a plan for next time you meet together, even if that's only online. There is real value in celebrating the positive times in your life as an Early Career Researcher. We all know that sharing the times when you are rejected will improve that experience. Similarly, celebrating the good times will give you more impetus to keep pushing through the down times. Extending this positive feeling to your co-authors, or those in your laboratory will always be appreciated.

Remember to make sure that all of your co-authors have a copy of the accepted version of the manuscript. Sometimes referred to as a **postprint**, you and your co-authors should submit this to your institutional repository so that the article can be reached as Green Open Access by anyone who is interested in reading it. Another option if your library does not have a repository is to use an Open Source service like Share Your Paper (shareyourpaper.org). Note that when self archiving, you will need to use the publisher's DOI in order to make your manuscript findable.

At the same time as your manuscript is accepted, or shortly thereafter, the publisher (if you are using a traditional style publisher model) will tell you when you can expect to receive the proofs.

20.1 Take your time with proofs

The next step in the publishing process, once your paper has been accepted, is that it will go for type setting. Depending on the journal and the publisher, this process can proceed in several ways. Typically you will receive a notification that your paper proofs are ready and that you need to check and return them within 48 hours.

DOI: 10.1201/9781003220886-20

135

Some journals may have an additional **copy editing** (also known as sub-editing) step. This is essentially an extra step checking journal style, syntax, punctuation, spelling and grammatical consistency. The copy editor may be tasked with checking additional issues, like species names (taxonomic authorities), names of chemical compounds used, etc. All will check citations against literature cited, and check that literature cited is sufficient to link with CrossRef. Most journals that I have worked with roll copy editing and proofing into a single step.

If you haven't checked proofs before, then it is important that you read the instructions from the publishers, that come with the proofs, carefully. They should tell you exactly what to do and if you are unsure about anything then talk to your co-authors.

Typically the publishers will send you a set of queries (copy edits) that relate to your proofs. They always ask you to check every author's name and affiliation. Other typical errors are that there are citations in the text that are not in the references. Or that there's literature in the references that are not cited.

The process of checking the proofs is very important. Errors can creep in during the type setting stage. Equally, copy editors can get it wrong, and you should read the text very carefully to make sure that errors have not been introduced. Pay special attention to the tables, table legends and figure legends.

You may also have the opportunity to change the size or orientation of figures, especially if it looks like they are not well presented in the proof. If the journal prints into columns, they may choose to put your figure in one column instead of across two. Another option is to have your figure in landscape across the whole page. Journals are generally pushed for space and so may refuse some requests for more room for larger figures. But you might get lucky if you make a good case.

Although the proofs are the responsibility of the corresponding author, it's good to get as many eyes on them as possible in order to spot any possible errors. Some journals let you know when proofs are likely to arrive, in which case it's a good idea to alert your co-authors and ask them whether they are prepared to look at them within that temporal window. I usually suggest that you make all your own corrections first before sending them around. Worst is for everyone to make their own corrections independently, as you'll have to put them all onto one set of proofs, and everyone is likely to spot some of the same errors.

Many publishers want proofs back in a hurry (typically 48 hours). If you don't have the confidence to correct proofs yourself, or cannot pass it around your co-authors within this deadline, then you can simply write back and ask for an extended deadline for your proofs. It is important to get it right, and much better than having to correct the paper later.

It is important that you make any corrections needed on the proofs. They are important to get right because once the proofs are submitted and the Version of Record is produced, any changes that you may want to make will require an official correction in the form of a separate publication.

Probably the easiest way of doing proofs is to print them out and go through them with a pencil first. This allows you to take your time and you're more likely to spot errors this way than on the screen. However, some publishers will require you to submit proofs in an online system (effectively working with their LaTeX document). You should still have an opportunity to print and take your time with the proofs though, and these systems do allow for this.

Sometimes, there are a lot of problems with proofs, and you may not have the confidence that the publishers will make all the corrections as indicated. In this case, you should ask to see another round of proofs before committing. Most publishers will happily send you a second round of proofs.

20.2   The DOI for your paper

The Digital Object Identifier (DOI) is an international standard (ISO) unique character string to identify physical, digital or abstract objects. The DOI is a 'persistent identifier' or 'permalink' which means that it remains unchanged even if the document itself changes location. For example, if the society that owns the journal changes their publisher, the DOIs of all content remain with the same documents even when they leave the old publisher's website. This means that although the publisher will provide a link to their website, and you may have your own repository with a link to your paper, you should rather use the DOI as the link to give out to everyone.

When you cite the DOI, don't take it apart, but provide the full link. For example, `https://doi.org/10.1242/jeb.233031` should never be abbreviated to 10.1242/jeb.233031 or doi.org/10.1242/jeb.233031.

You will note that old DOIs look different (they used http instead of https protocol, and typically have dx.doi.org addresses), but you should not edit the start of their address, but leave them. For example: `http://dx.doi.org/10.1098/rspb.2018.2528`

Sometimes your article may acquire several DOIs, for example from the publisher and from the preprint server. Sites like figshare and ResearchGate, assign different DOIs to content uploaded to their platforms. These are DOIs but they're assigned by DataCite, another DOI registration agency. The different registration agencies provide different services that relate to DOIs and their associated metadata (from construction to the movie industry), and have different requirements for their member organisations. To prevent ambiguity, you should always use the DOI associated with the Version of Record. The biggest player registering content in scholarly output is CrossRef.

There are still some journals that do not issue DOIs. But the cost associated with adding DOIs by small publishers is changing, and so it is likely that in future a DOI will be associated with all scholarly output.

DOIs are extremely useful as you can usually click on an active link DOI and go straight to the article in question. Therefore it is well worth adding the DOI to your references if you can. Most reference databases will do this automatically, but if they don't pick up the DOI for some reason, then it's worth adding it yourself. Some journals will demand it, while others have yet to come around to how useful they are.

However, DOIs cannot replace references, otherwise we'd need to be able to click on every link all the time, and couldn't read any paper without a connection to the internet. It's still really useful to be able to read a formatted reference at the end of a paper.

Publishers normally deposit DOIs and other metadata (authors' names and addresses, publication dates, title, licence, funders, etc.) around the time the article is published online. This is called content registration. This is not just for articles, but also preprints, conference proceedings, books, book chapters, peer reviews and more can all have their content registered with CrossRef. The standardisation of this metadata means that not only is it possible to immediately find your article (the DOI is a link), but all of the metadata associated with it can be cross-referenced. This is of great help to funders, for example, who can look up all the products that their funding has produced without having to contact all of the people that they funded.

20.2.1   DOI tools

If you can't find the DOI for an article that you want to cite, then there is this very useful online software that will provide the DOI if there is one for every reference you enter: `doi.crossref.org/simpleTextQuery` or use the CrossRef Metadata Search: search.crossref.org/references

There's an equally useful database that provides BibTex for DOIs that you enter: doi2bib.org

20.3 Add your paper to your ORCID account

The ORCID (orcid.org) number was devised to provide a common platform for authors to curate, and now some journals and funding authorities won't allow you to submit or apply without one. This helps when there are authors with common (or even identical) names. As an NGO dedicated to helping scientists ascribe credit for their work, it should be supported. ORCID will also help prevent author fraud (see Part I).

If you added your ORCID number to the metadata when you uploaded your manuscript, your ORCID record should be updated automatically (through CrossRef) when the DOI of your article appears online. Inside your ORCID account, you can grant permission for CrossRef to update the records automatically, otherwise you will need to log onto ORCID from time to time and approve changes suggested there. Alternatively, you can add works to your ORCID record via CrossRef Metadata Search.

Be careful not to create duplicate accounts, and make your ORCID available to your collaborators so that they aren't left guessing at your identity when it comes to submitting a paper. ORCID allows you to create some useful links for your website or a QR code for adding to posters and presentations. If you find you have a duplicated account, it is simple to remove it (see here[1]).

20.4 Once you have a publication date

Once your paper is published you have an opportunity to publicise it yourself. There are lots of different ways to do this, see the next chapters. Some funders and institutions will want to know about press worthy publications before they are published, so that they can prepare a press release.

20.5 On the day you publish

This is a great opportunity to contact all the people who helped you in your study and send them a PDF of your paper. The easiest way to do this is to go

---

[1]https://support.orcid.org/hc/en-us/articles/360006896634

to the acknowledgements section and write an email that includes everyone that is mentioned in the acknowledgements. Write them a nice email in which you thank them for their help and explain briefly the significance of the paper.

It is a very good idea to keep all of these people informed about your publication as soon as it is published. You really want people in your network to hear about it from you first and not from somebody else. This includes contacting any authorities that have issued permits. You may also want to contact funders.

21

Writing a press release

Many of the aspects to do with writing a press release are similar to those needed when writing a popular article. Try to make your text newsworthy. Remember that journalists are looking for new things, that's why it's called 'The News'. Your press release must be about something that has happened recently. There's no point in writing a press release about a paper that was published six or nine months ago. It's very unlikely that you'll find anyone interested in writing something after that amount of time.

Here are 10 simple steps to consider when writing your press release:

1. **Choose your hook**. The paper that you wrote may have several important findings. You are going to need to choose one easy to understand finding for your media release. It's usually quite simple to decide; take the thing that would most impress your Auntie Fanny.

2. **Write your headline**. Like choosing a good journal title or a popular story title the headline should try to encapsulate the study perhaps with a witty angle. Don't make it too long, eight to ten words at most. Most importantly your headline should connect with a wide and general readership. There's no need to get too fond of your headline because, if they take your story, news outlets are likely to want to write their own.

3. **Crafting the first paragraph** is important. You need to sum up the study together with the finding. Even if your reader only reads the first paragraph they should have an understanding of what you've done and found. This first paragraph should not be longer than 30 words.

4. In the second paragraph, you should **state who you are and where you are from**, both geographically and the name of your institute. Here you need to concentrate on getting across the information on why you're finding is interesting. A typical second paragraph might read:

Dr Frankella Smith from FitsSimon's University found a new species of woodlouse when bending down to tie her shoelaces last

DOI: 10.1201/9781003220886-21

month. She published her findings today in the journal *Cobblers'
Oniscids.*

---

5. In the next two paragraphs you should simply explain more about
   the background to your story and why the finding is interesting.
   Don't be tempted to deviate from the hook that you've chosen. After
   reading these two paragraphs your reader should be able to answer
   the question: So what?
6. Finally sum up your finding with a quote from you, the author.
   Either use the quote to emphasise the study results, or you can try
   and humanise your findings. This means a way of connecting with
   the reader, especially if you feel that the rest of your text won't:

"I never expected to find such a pretty woodlouse on my shoe",
said Frankclla. "I was flabbergasted when it turned out to be
new to science."

---

7. Include your name and contact details of the person that the press
   should contact in order to find out more about the story.
8. Give the full citation to the paper with all the author names and
   the journal name plus a link so that any journalist can find the full
   text online.
9. Include one or two photographs or relevant graphics that the press
   can use. If they are not taken by you then make sure that you have
   permission to use them. If you can, include a picture of the study
   organism, or even better of you with the study organism.
10. Seek feedback. Send your press release to your university's press
    office and ask for feedback. Those are the professionals and they
    should be able to help you.

Of course, the better your press release is, the more likely it will be that people
will write about it. Remember that it also matters a lot about the subject
of your paper. The media are likely to be far more interested if your work is
on dolphin communication than if you are writing about isopod appendages
(just like your Auntie Fanny). Having said this, never be put off just because
your organism or system isn't cute and cuddly. Try asking your non-academic
friends about the newsworthiness of your press release and see what they say.

22

Why write a popular article?

There are many reasons why it is important to communicate science beyond your own discipline and into the wider public forum. Primary among these is that in a civic society based on decisions made on the basis of science, it is our responsibility as scientists to make sure that we make the findings of our work, upon which basis political decisions are made, understood to the widest of audiences. I do not mean that we are sharing science pejoratively to an ignorant public, but instead as equals in our collective scientific society. We share with a wider public in the same way that we share with those who are used to reading a well-reasoned newspaper article, or listening to an informed political debate. By sharing our work, we help affirm that decisions should be made objectively, and we make the most important connection by reaching out to the rest of our society and to join them in the scientific project.

Here are some extra reasons why communicating by writing a popular article might be right for you:

- Inform tax-payers who funded research of what you found
- Increase the profile of your work and you as a researcher
- Reach other researchers (who also read popular articles)
- Reach other stakeholders like practitioners or policy makers
- Open more doors to other potentially cross-disciplinary work
- Gain new insights into how your work appears to the general public
- Public communication is a key part of social responsibility, quickly becoming a key aspect of an academic career
- Maintaining and furthering the Scientific Project

The sooner that you come to terms with the need to communicate your work more widely, the more comfortable you will be when you are contacted by a reporter, a vlogger or someone from TV or radio.

DOI: 10.1201/9781003220886-22

22.1   Here's a quick guide on how to get started writing a popular article.

Just like any writing project, there is no one way to write a popular article. I provide the following advice in order to get you started. You are, of course, free to write however you think your work will be best understood and appreciated.

What's the hook? Your popular article will not be the same as your paper. You should plan to have a single fact or message that you want the public to walk away with after reading your article. This is likely to be the same as the main result in your paper.

When composing your article, you need to be single minded about achieving the understanding of your hook. The article cannot take any side roads or distractions, but must stick to the main point. Once that's done, provide the 'so what' that allows the reader to see the bigger picture, and maybe where you would go next.

Don't get complex or technical If your whole article hinges on something technical, you might have to start by explaining it simply. If you can't easily explain it, then this is probably the wrong subject for a popular article. Don't worry about leaving out (what might be to you) key details, you can always refer the reader to your article if they want to know more.

Always refer to your published work Make sure that you always have some reference to your work that's published. Provide a hyperlink, but preferably give the full citation. Be aware that news items count towards the altmetrics of your article, so be sure to link it correctly.

Pictures, videos and even sound files These are great to help readers engage with your work. Try to choose images that tell the story with the same information as you have in your article. If you don't have any, then try asking your co-authors, and then try to remember for the next project that you need to collect these when doing your research as it really helps when publicising your work.

23

Altmetrics from traditional and social media

In recent years, more emphasis has been placed on the way that scientists communicate their work. Many institutions now consider the degree to which scientists communicate their work as one of several key performance areas on which they are judged. Because administrators are always looking for simple solutions to evaluate the work of many different types of academics, commercial solutions to measuring the degree of communication for each publication have sprung up. The most ubiquitous of these in Biological Sciences are **'altmetrics'** (Priem et al., 2012): alternative metrics that aim to measure activity on the internet through social media (e.g. Twitter, Facebook), online reference managers (e.g. Mendeley, Zotero), blogs and traditional media outlets. Because of the immediacy of these activities, altmetrics tend to accumulate much faster than traditional citations, giving a near immediate impression of the interest generated in an article.

A prominent company producing altmetrics for many biological journals is Altmetric (www.altmetric.com). The whirls they produce, known as 'Altmetric badges' are coloured to show the proportions of different media that have been scraped from the web (Figure 23.1). Although Altmetric are widely used, the calculation of their impact score is not transparent. For example, in March 2021 they changed the weighting of their impact score so that Tweets (which were weighted at 86.9% of the score) lost 75% of their effect (Anderson, 2021). They did this without an announcement or the knowledge of their staff. Verifying the calculation of scores doesn't always add up, and I've noticed that even their web crawling news coverage can be hit and miss.

A better option would be an open source tool to track altmetrics data transparently. Such tools have been developed (e.g Paperbuzz: paperbuzz.org and ImpactStory: profiles.impactstory.org), but at the time of writing these initiatives are unfunded and adrift.

In Biological Sciences, there is a traditional bias in media coverage towards species with higher charisma (Bonnet et al., 2002; Ducarme et al., 2013). This means that if you work on whales or roses, your work is likely to generate much higher altmetrics than if you conduct equivalent work on phasmids or grasses. Traditional media is starting to make an effort away from only reporting on science with charismatic species, but they are driven by a public with insatiable demand for kittens and flowers.

DOI: 10.1201/9781003220886-23

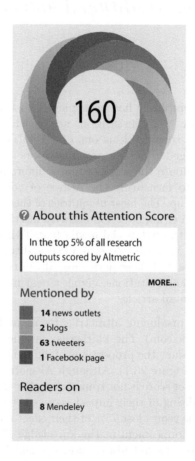

FIGURE 23.1: The whirl output for a single paper from an Altmetrics analysis. In this example, a paper by Baxter-Gilbert et al. (2020) was covered by many Tweets, news outlets, some blogs and a Facebook mention. Altmetric provides an overall score, but different types of mentions are not equal, so a news outlet is awarded a higher score than a Tweet. Although this paper did not garner interest due to being a charismatic species, the story was of general interest to the public as it centred on island dwarfism. Reproduced with permission.

There is a lot that you can do to improve the level of your altmetrics, like writing a popular article or a press release. As communication is becoming so important in the careers of scientists, then I'd suggest that you remain aware of altmetrics and how they are used by your institution. Be aware of how to influence and increase your score. For example, if you and your friends tweet about your article, make sure that there is a live link to the article on the publisher's website. Similarly, if you are contacted by a news outlet about some of your research, you can insist that they place a link to your paper in their article. If the Altmetric scraper cannot find coverage on your paper, you can inform them at www.altmetric.com/about-our-data/our-sources.

Part IV

Further challenges in academia

24

Is Open Access good?

Open access appears to be a great initiative that acknowledges that everything should be free to view. Neither scientists nor the public that fund them should be barred from accessing the knowledge that is produced. What could be wrong with Open Access? Many people have written a great deal on what has gone wrong, and what I provide here (and elsewhere in this book) is not the last word as this is a dynamic topic that is changing all the time.

24.1   So what is Open Access?

I have covered the many different kinds of Open Access (OA) elsewhere in this book (see part II). Here I concentrate on the fiscal implication of OA. Someone needs to pay for the work done. Who should pay and how?

The principle of Open Access is something that is easy to appreciate, and lies very much at the heart at the movement from closed to open science. Some history is appropriate when we discuss Open Access, because the movement started as a genuine attempt to change the publishing model for the better (see key texts including those by Poynder, 2019, 2020). Hopefully in the future this experiment will be seen as a success. In the meantime, Open Access has been employed by publishers as a way in which they can earn large amounts of additional income. The story of *PLOS ONE* is useful to see how this change came about.

24.1.1   *PLOS ONE*

The Public Library of Science (PLOS) started soon after the turn of the new millennium, primarily as a concern to the problems with peer review that are highlighted elsewhere in this book. This really was a new experiment in publishing, that was to radically alter the publishing model in the 21st century, and in only ten years, *PLOS ONE* became the world's biggest journal. The idea was to do away with all the normal waiting times in publishing, and to

DOI: 10.1201/9781003220886-24

have articles published immediately online, and without any charges associated with accessing them: Open Access. At the time, this was all fairly radical, and it became very successful with a large amount of interest from scientists who submitted their articles to PLOS journals. But the founders were frustrated that they were rejecting a lot of papers that were technically good, but not selected as they were not novel, or did not significantly advance their field. In 2006, PLOS dreamt up a new journal to take all of these technically sound manuscripts, and this was the birth of *PLOS ONE*.

From the outset, *PLOS ONE* was not interested in acquiring any Impact Factor. Instead, it was mostly interested in taking technically sound manuscripts irrespective of their results. This meant that reviewers for *PLOS ONE* were (and still are) asked to assess the technical soundness of a manuscript, and not to judge the 'value' of the results. The original idea was that reviews should be post publication, through comments made on the website after the publications were posted. The initial review then, was simply meant as a preliminary check for technical soundness. This was again a radical departure from the publishing norm by the PLOS group, when many other journals were still rejecting manuscripts that had no faults other than they were not attractive to editors. *PLOS ONE* was opened to accept all such manuscripts, effectively doing away with publication bias. As you might imagine, at a time when academics were under pressure to 'publish or perish', rejections were plentiful, and so manuscripts quickly found their way to *PLOS ONE*. Because *PLOS ONE* was also Open Access, its papers received an extra boost of citations through visibility, and ironically after five years it found that it had an Impact Factor to rival some of the journals whose rejections it was picking up. This meant that more and more scientists started submitting to *PLOS ONE* as their journal of choice, mostly because it was publishing Open Access.

PLOS ONE became the world's biggest scientific journal, and in 2013 it published 32,058 papers (Davies, 2019). It's worth taking a moment to do the arithmetic on the income that PLOS received for these at > USD 1000 per article (so it seems inconceivable that they could ever make a loss). By this time, other academic publishers had noticed the rocketing ascent of *PLOS ONE* and had responded by starting their own 'no Impact Factor' journals that could be fed by the rejection piles of journals already in their stables. Notable among these was *Scientific Reports* from the Nature Publishing Group which started in 2011 with 208 papers, and after 7 years ramping up to nearly 20,000 papers in 2018. For whatever reason, the Impact Factor of *Scientific Reports* is roughly double that of *PLOS ONE* for around the same article processing charge (APC), drawing far more researchers in. During this same period, since 2013, a great many such examples of 'no Impact Factor' journals that accept any article that is technically sound began to appear. They are not only the general behemoths like *PLOS ONE* and *Scientific Reports*, but you will find that even niche journals that make significant numbers of rejections of technically sound papers have their own version that they will offer to you in the same email that informs you of a rejection from their flagship journal.

The bottom line, from this story of PLOS ONE, the highly innovative journal with an attempt to fundamentally change the publishing landscape, is that this is exactly what it did. However, mainstream publishers saw a massive and untapped market and decided not to call these new entities 'no impact factor' journals, or even the 'rejection pile,' but placed them under the Open Access banner.

As a result of the PLOS ONE success, there was a bandwagon movement to Open Access. Now the scientists pay for making their own content open for anyone to read. They pay a one-off fee to the publishers to typeset the manuscript and host it on their site without a paywall. Prices start from USD 1000 and go up to around USD 12,000. Prices often increase with the Impact Factor of the journal (Gray, 2020; Mekonnen et al., 2021), although the costs involved to the publisher remain static. Actual costs of publishing a research paper in 2021 have been estimated as between USD 200 and USD 1000 (for the most prestigious journals with a rejection rate >90%) (Grossmann and Brembs, 2021).

24.2   So does that mean that OA journals are now free?

Mostly no. The majority OA model (hybrid OA) means that a minority of articles in these journals are free, but the universities are expected to subscribe to those same journals at ever increasing prices because much of the rest of the content is still behind the paywall. This is because most authors cannot afford to pay the fees charged by the journals (although some countries now have this payment as mandatory – cOAlition S (www.coalition-s.org), they and their scientists are still in a minority). There are some journals that are entirely Open Access (gold OA and diamond OA). These are (almost) exclusively online and have never been part of traditional packages that university libraries spend so much of their budget on. Hence the fact that they are entirely free to read does not impact library budgets. 'Transformative publishing agreements' (Janicke Hinchliffe, 2019) are a new model discussed later in the book, estimated to cost two to three times as much as the traditional publishing model (Poynder, 2020; Table 28.1).

But paying for open access has not reduced the cost of access to scientific journals for libraries. This cost constantly goes up. For Hybrid OA, we pay for much of this content not twice but thrice (Buranyi, 2017)!

You, as an Early Career Researcher, are in one of the best positions to do something about the change from closed to open science. Currently, diamond OA journals are a very small and quite unusual component of the publishing scene. But it is totally possible for these to become mainstream using initiatives like the overlay journal system. The current dynamic will only change when academics submitting their manuscripts change from for-profit publishers to other models. The power is literally in your choice of where to send your manuscript.

24.3   The wicked problem

Publishing has become very expensive for scientists and their funders. In parts of the world these costs are preventing some scientists from publishing where they want to. In richer nations, funders are now allocating increasing resources away from science and towards publishing. Publishing metrics are driving the hiring and promotion of scientists globally (Part IV), and competition for these are increasingly associated with fraud and misconduct. Choice of study subjects are leaning more towards publishing content with important metrics, than the acquisition of knowledge for the societies that are funding it. There is also the suggestion that some publishers have begun to capture the academic workflow with a view to selling associated data (Brembs et al., 2021). We, as scientists, are allowing this to happen, and even paying for the privilege. Together with our institutions, funders and governments, we perpetuate the dominance of publishing in our scientific domain.

A wicked problem is one that is not only complex, but lacks clarity (with respect to solutions) or a way to scientifically test and study it. According to Rittel and Webber (1973), there are ten important characteristics, all of which are met by the ongoing situation in academic publishing. There are multiple stakeholders in our wicked problem, and they include our employers, our funders (political and societal), our peers as well as the gatekeepers and societies that police the system. It is up to you to be aware of the options and become part of a solution that benefits science.

As scientists, we need to go back to our core concerns around **the scientific method: rigour, independence, transparency and reproducibility**. We need to persuade our institutions that our core concerns are what we should be measured by, and that the new range of Open Science tools be used to determine the extent to which we live up to our scientific values. Getting jobs, tenure and grants should be based on our Open Science credentials instead of the publishing industry serving Impact Factor and other publishing metrics.

24.3.1 Choosing open source for Open Science

These days 'printing' really means hosting electronic pdfs only, as there's very little paper that's actually printed. The layout from the manuscript (most often written in a word processing document) into a formatted pdf takes skill and talent. Today it is possible to use free software, like R Markdown (Xie, Allaire & Grolemund, 2018), to write papers that can quickly and easily be made into any sophisticated layout using LaTeX, the same language used by the publishers. Current models suggest that this way of formatting costs as little as USD 10 per paper (Grossmann & Brembs, 2021). Many journals allow submission of articles already formatted this way. Some publishers are buying these tools (e.g. Overleaf, Mendeley, Peerwith, Authorea, etc.) as part of the academic workflow that could be used as spyware (Brembs et al., 2021).

There are large costs associated with placing journals on platforms that allow for the dissemination, peer review and archiving, all essential for academic journals. Currently, there is no open source equivalent to a big publishing company that hosts hundreds or thousands of academic journals. But this does not mean that it is not possible. Once the investment has been made to set up such a platform, adding another 10 or 20 journals comes at practically no cost.

24.4 Making the change

My message, throughout this book, has been that the tools to make the shift from closed to open science are available to us now (Brembs et al., 2021). In my view, scholarly publishing is incompatible with all OA models except diamond OA, which necessitates a movement away from current publishers and back to the academic domain (see Fuchs & Sandoval, 2013; Brembs et al., 2021). There is nothing to stop us changing the system other than the need to act collectively. Indeed, there is an imperative to change the system as soon as we can to avoid academic capture.

Scholarly societies offer an excellent opportunity to organise and act collectively. Some societies still dictate terms to publishers (e.g. The British Ecological Society) and they have the power to finish their contracts and move their journals to new diamond Open Access formats, using tools such as overlay journals. In turn, they have to give up the income that their for-profit publishers supply. This does not mean that they would lose all income, they would still have membership funds and conferences. But there would be a loss of some of the comfort that they have become used to, making giving up hard to do. But societies need to carry out the wish of their members, and I would suggest that there are more members that would benefit from diamond Open Access to society journals, than currently see any benefit in the payouts from deals with for-profit publishers.

25

How to conduct peer review

Here I will assume that you have been given a peer review assignment. If you aren't getting asked to do any reviews, there are some suggestions on how to get started in Part I.

Most modern journals provide reviewers with a guideline on how they expect peer review to be done. I encourage you to read the specific instructions that are given by journals on how to conduct peer review for them. There are also a number of excellent blogs to read about peer review (including this one: Raff, 2013). A systematic assessment of these requirements in biomedical journals has been undertaken by Glonti et al. (2019) and Eve et al. (2021). These accounts are worth dipping into for an overview on the different sorts of statements that peer reviewers come up with. You can see, in the quantitative analysis of Eve et al. (2021), that the overwhelming number of comments are those of skilled critics. This study also makes it clear that the role of the peer reviewer is often ambiguous and that reviews are not consistent in what they deliver.

Essentially peer reviewers are tasked with determining whether or not the manuscript is credible.

- Could the study be repeated?
- Are the methods legitimate in order to produce the results provided
- Are the results sufficient to respond to the hypothesis posed?
- Can it be improved?
- Is the content of the manuscript appropriate to the journal?
- Does the experimental design contain sufficient controls?
- Did the authors try and stretch the implications of their results beyond the credibility of the findings?

Once you have conducted your peer review, you can log it on Publons (www.publons.com) in order to get credit later on. Publons also carries your publication output and citations (tied to Web of Science), so can be a useful way of keep track of your own productivity for reporting purposes (but see the section on Impact Factor).

DOI: 10.1201/9781003220886-25

25.1 Novelty or repeatability?

At the heart of scientific enquiry is that studies done should be repeatable, with the presumption that if they have been done in the same way they should achieve the same results (given the bounds of significance testing – see Forstmeier et al., 2017). Hence, you must examine and report on whether or not the study's materials and methods are sufficient for someone else to repeat the study. This appears to be surprisingly rare in peer review (at ~4% according to Eve et al., 2021). For some no impact journals, this technical soundness will be enough to allow them to pass peer review.

Many journals that aspire to increase their Impact Factor, ask for a comment on how novel the study is. This is a somewhat subjective question, as individuals have biased opinions of what constitutes something novel, noteworthy, of significance or of relevance to the audience of a particular journal. Hence, this is really going to be a point that you can decide based on your own understanding of the literature (remembering that you have been chosen because your opinion counts).

You can gain important insight into what is relevant, and what not, in peer review from the analysis of *PLOS ONE* reviews by Eve et al. (2021).

25.2 Parts of your review

Just as we discussed the different parts of a review when thinking about writing a rebuttal, here we discuss the same parts from the view of writing the review. I think that, in addition to reading this section, it is worth refreshing your memory about receiving peer review, when thinking about writing one.

25.2.1 A positive appraisal of the study

Summarising the study in your own words, to the tune of a single paragraph, is a useful way to start a review.

- It is usually positive being skewed towards what you understood, and what was well communicated.
- Concentrates the minds of reviewers, making them think about the whole manuscript (and not simply focussing on minutiae).
- Lets authors know exactly what came across (and by omission what didn't).

- Allows editors to contrast your understanding with what other reviewers contributed, as well as their own interpretation. Usually different people find different issues, but overall the impression should be broadly congruent.

If you have not understood everything, then you should concentrate on what you have understood to be reported in this section. Although this might set you up to produce a 'shit sandwich', this is not necessarily a bad thing.

25.2.2 Major comments

The next section concerns major positive and negative comments. Try to be even handed here. This is a place to point out any major short-falls of the manuscript, but it should also be used to point out where the authors have done a good job. You may need to resort to a list, where each major item gets it's own paragraph, but these may turn into sections if your reasoning takes longer.

For each major comment, give an example of what you mean with line numbers. These should be tangible points that you can tie down to things that are present in (or even missing from) the text. In this section, I would urge you to keep away from providing subjective statements (like 'I think...' or 'I feel...' or 'It seems to me...'). If you need to voice these feelings, then keep them for a final paragraph where you make it clear that these are impressions given by the manuscript to the reader.

25.2.3 Minor concerns

List these out under a new heading **Minor Comments** starting each one with a line number where it occurs. Figures and tables should receive their own comments (no line numbers required, but give the Figure or Table number).

25.3 The spirit of peer review

In their heart, a peer reviewer should be trying their best to improve the manuscript they read as much as they possibly can. This may simply represent an improvement in the way the text is worded. But it may also mean adding extra analyses or even experiments (within the bounds of reason).

As McPeek et al. (2009) put it, the golden rule of reviewing is to do unto others as you would have them do unto you. You could also read Baglini and

Parsons (2020), who provide some useful insight into how to remain neutral when making reviewer comments. Again, the emphasis is on being professional.

25.3.1   There are ethical considerations for reviewers

- Reviewers may not share manuscripts with other scientists unless specific permission is given by the editor.
- Similarly reviewers should not discuss the content of manuscripts that they are reviewing.
- Reviewers should not try to take the work presented in the manuscript and copy it for publication (i.e. do not steal the ideas).
- Reviews should be conducted within a reasonable time frame. No reviewer should hold on to a manuscript especially if they have a vested interest (like a rival study) in not seeing it published. This should have been declared as conflict of interest.
- Any other potential conflicts of interest, including those that might make you positively predisposed to the authors, should be declared.
- Reviewers should be aware of their own prejudices and biases and not bring them through to the review process.
- You must decide whether or not to sign your review. Given the opportunity ~43% of reviewers will provide published open reviews (Wang et al., 2016). Would you want your reviewer to sign?

In essence these ethical issues are overcome when reviewers conform to transparency. In order to facilitate transparency in peer review, Parker et al. (2018) have produced a checklist that I encourage you to use if and when you are asked to conduct a review.

25.3.2   Remain objective and rational

Your job as a reviewer will be to remain objective about the manuscript that you are reading, pointing out its merits and problems without succumbing to bias. Forming your own world view of your topic within the Biological Sciences does mean that you likely need a form of directionally motivated reasoning. For example, this is why you decide to investigate one hypothesis before another, or feel that one line of investigation is more salient to your area than another. These could be made through observations or experiences that you have had during your research, or they may come from schools of thought within your discipline. But it is important that you remain **intellectually honest**, to allow others to hold alternative, valid arguments. Just as it is important in your own work that you are always prepared to accept the null hypothesis as readily as you do the alternative hypothesis. One lesson revealed from reading lots of peer reviews is that reviewers find it hard to remain centred using accuracy motivated reasoning, all too often resorting to attacking the authors or their experiment (Eve et al., 2021). Your principle task is to remain intellectually honest in your review, such that you can point out faulty arguments without perverting the direction that the authors planned to take. Equally, it is important that the authors acknowledge alternative viewpoints, but not to the extent that they should be made to abandon their own interpretation.

Psychologists have argued that as humans we cannot be expected to be rational, and that we are not particularly good at being objective. But this doesn't mean that we shouldn't try, and it also means that by being aware of the potential problems in peer review, we are in a better position to learn how to avoid them.

Write every review as if it will be public. Ask yourself whether every statement that you make can be backed up either by other references in the literature, or with line numbers corresponding to erroneous logic on the part of the authors. Although this strategy is not guaranteed to produce an unbiased review, it will be an intellectually honest way to approach the manuscript. If you have the choice, then do make your review public to hold with the Open Communication ethos of Open Science.

25.3.3 Remember to accentuate the positive

Peer review is often thought of as being brutal, where anonymous reviewers have the opportunity to vent their darkest thoughts. Certainly, there are plenty of reviewers who are unprofessional in what they say (Eve et al., 2021; Hyland and Jiang, 2020). When conducting peer review, you have the opportunity to be one of the goodies. You can point out where the authors have done due diligence, in their experimental design, reporting, analyses, etc. This is likely to benefit the authors far more than pointing out only the problems – especially those that cannot be fixed.

25.3.4 How long should your review be?

Quite simply, you need to write enough until you have reviewed the manuscript. The length of peer review varies wildly, from 200 characters to 43,000 (likely more than the article itself), according to Eve et al. (2021). The distribution peaks between 2000 and 4000 characters, and this should be a good guide.

If you submit your review to a service like publons (publons.com), you can compare the lengths of your reviews which get charted against those of the 'average reviewer', and I would suggest that you should aim to keep your reviews around average length, using any extra words to help the authors. There's no point in just writing extra words to increase your character count!

25.3.5 What to do if you suspect fraud?

The Committee on Publication Ethics (www.publicationethics.org) (COPE) has published some useful flowcharts to guide reviewers who suspect fraud in manuscripts they are reading. A list of these is provided in Part IV.

25.3.6 Further help with conducting peer review

A number of publishers and academic institutes have provided online resources to help train those undertaking peer review (e.g. ACS Reviewer Lab; Publons Academy; Nature Masterclass). Remember that these are suggestions, and should provide sufficient instruction to get you started. Not all journals ask the same of their reviewers, and so instructions may vary. Your review should follow the recommendations provided by the journal that you are providing the review for.

26

The problems with peer review

There is already a lot covering peer review in this book, and I have placed this chapter last not because it is the least significant, potentially it is the most significant, but because I think that it is important that you appreciate exactly what peer review is, and experience it from both sides, before you begin to consider the problems with the peer review system.

At the heart of the problems with peer review is that individual humans are themselves biased. Because peer review relies on a small number of individuals providing their assessment of a manuscript, it is quite likely that these biases might align, and that the manuscript is rejected along those lines, rather than being considered along purely objective lines. This likelihood of aligned prejudices comes about because the pool of people that conduct peer review in Biological Sciences, and in many other disciplines, is mostly white, western (i.e. Europe and North America) and male. These people hold a very similar cultural set of biases.

Some people have argued that peer review is untested and that the effects are uncertain (Jefferson et al., 2002). Perhaps more worryingly, studies designed to test peer review (by deliberately sending out manuscripts with errors) have shown that most reviewers are unable to find all errors and some find none (Rothwell and Martyn, 2000).

For example, if peer review was effective, then reviews of grant applications should closely align with the productivity of grants given. Fang et al. (2016) found that percentile scores awarded by peer review of NIH grant applications were poor at predicting the the productivity of >100,000 grants awarded.

Essentially, the major problem with peer review is that it is conducted by humans, and that like humans in societies everywhere, reviewers tend to have their own set of biases. The following sections should have given you some idea about the frailties of the peer review system.

DOI: 10.1201/9781003220886-26

26.1 Upsetting comments

I think that the reason why we find review comments so harsh is usually because we put so much effort into the writing process that it feels very personal whenever we receive criticism. Indeed, I think that there might be a correlation between how much effort you put in and how harsh the reviewers' comments seem. Another study suggests that authors consider the competence of their reviewers to be closely aligned to the editorial decision (Drvenica et al., 2019). Just be aware that this is normal. Remember that the reviewers are humans, and they have sat down and given freely of their own time to read your work. The most important thing to be aware of is that all they had was what you had written. No background information, and possibly no information about the species or the system involved. They will be experts at some level, but perhaps not the type you might expect. Importantly, the editor asked them because they thought that their opinion would be of importance in helping them make their decision on your paper. This means that you also need to respect their opinion and comments, even if you don't agree with them or find them to be offensive, arrogant or even rude. Remember also that some apparent rudeness may just be a reviewer who has a sense of humour that you don't understand. There are lots of examples of this at ShitMyReviewersSay (shitmyreviewerssay.tumblr.com). So no matter what you think of each comment, you should respond to it in a professional and courteous manner that shows that you are a professional scientist.

Why do scientists make disparaging or unprofessional remarks to their colleagues in peer review? Whenever two or three scientists get together, you hear tales of recent woes associated with peer review. The retelling of such stories is all part of the collective, cathartic unburdening of what can be a traumatic experience especially when we put so much effort into each piece of work (see Hyland and Jiang, 2020). Reading through a lot of these reviewers' comments, I can see that there is an attempt at humour. This humour is not appreciated by those who receive the reviews. Perhaps I understand the humour, because I also come from that same culture that dominates STEM, but that is not understood or even recognised as humour by others. Writing humorous reviews is unprofessional, especially if it is used to accentuate negative aspects. Needless to say, we could all do without unprofessional reviews.

26.2   *Ad hominem* attacks

One of the shocking results of a very large study of peer review of *PLOS ONE* articles is the large number of comments that are written directly attacking the authors as a group or personally (i.e. *ad hominem* attacks, see Eve et al., 2021). This should not happen. Reviewers should confine their objective comments to the work and its presentation. However, this is an aspect of peer review where authors (especially the corresponding and leading authors) will need to acquire a thick skin, because unprofessional comments are made to people across gender and racial groupings, but especially towards traditionally underrepresented groups (Silbiger and Stubler, 2019). Sadly, these same groups feel that such comments disproportionately impact their productivity and career advancement (Silbiger and Stubler, 2019). Reading comments that are sent to other authors can be cathartic as these allow you to see that everyone receives such negative comments. ShitMyReviewersSay is a good source of these, or see Eve et al. (2021), or Silbiger and Stubler (2019). When *ad hominem* attacks are made, it would be good if editors openly and explicitly identified these as **bad behaviour**. It would certainly improve the understanding of authors if editors intervened when such *ad hominem* attacks are made. This would not necessarily involve deleting these comments, but directing authors to ignore the same.

Why do academics make all of these terrible comments? I can't pretend to know the answer for all of the cases, but I can speak from personal experience. Time is at a premium, and time spent reading and reviewing manuscripts tends to be quality time – best when it is quiet and uninterrupted. If these manuscripts are not of a quality that will pass peer review (i.e. will be rejected), then this feels like an abuse of professional time – especially when editors should have spotted the same mistake in their first reading. Editors that fail to see manuscripts that should be rejected do the reviewers a dis-service by increasing the amount of work for everyone (more people and more time is involved). Resentment and frustration may follow on the part of reviewers that manifests itself in the form of *ad hominem* attacks.

26.3   Demonstrated biases in peer review

Although Table 26.1 shows that many kinds of bias have been explicitly demonstrated, that's certainly not their limit. Given that over 280 biases have already been catalogued (I encourage you to look through the online catalogue: www.catalogofbias.org), many more different types of bias are likely to exist in peer review. Let's not forget that our biases have evolved because they are very useful. They exist as a way of shortcutting exhaustive decision making based on random variables. But maybe peer review needs some more of this. And perhaps that means that I should be tolerant when I'm asked to review an economics journal, as these folk clearly weren't exhibiting any biases associated with economists when they picked me (see Chapter 18).

TABLE 26.1: There are as many biases in peer review as there are humans that conduct them. This table demonstrates some of the biases that have been proven in studies.

Bias for which there is evidence	Study demonstrating bias
Against female authors	Tregenza (2002); Manlove and Belou (2018); Fox and Paine (2019); Budden et al. (2008); Morgan et al. (2018); Hagan et al. (2020)
Against female reviewers	Helmer et al. (2017); Fox et al. (2019)
Towards author reputation, favouring acceptance of manuscripts despite poor reviews	Bravo et al. (2018); Okike et al. (2016)
Towards authors from more prestigious institutions, also called prestige bias	Ceci and Peters (1982); Travis and Collins (1991); Garfunkel et al. (1994); Tomkins et al. (2017); Manlove and Belou (2018) ; Lee et al. (2013)
Nationality and language bias	Song et al. (2000); Lee et al. (2013); Manlove and Belou (2018); Nuñez and Amano (2021); Link (1998)
Confirmation bias (the tendency for journals and reviewers to favour significant results)	Mahoney (1977); Fanelli (2010); Fanelli (2012); see Part I[1]
Publication bias (the literature contains a bias in published results)	Jennions and Møller (2002); Munafò et al. (2007); Van Dongen (2011); Franco et al. (2014); Fanelli et al. (2017); Sánchez-Tójar et al. (2018); see Part IV

Perhaps the biggest problem facing those who wish to reform the peer review system is that it all starts with editors who are choosing reviewers. Those editors themselves have their own inherent biases. When they look for reviewers, they are likely to sample from within their own group of peers who have the same biases. Interestingly, bias (in general) is more easily perceived by early career scientists (Zvereva and Kozlov, 2021). My experience is that soliciting reviews from people that I don't know and have no connection with (are outside

---

[1] `transparency.html`

of my field) are more likely to fail – they will say no, or they won't reply to the request (see Perry et al., 2012). This is even for academics that are publishing within the same area.

Editors are the people who select reviewers, and inspection of most editorial boards will reveal that they reflect the same biases found in peer review. That is, editorial boards are mostly made up of white men from Europe and North America. Rectifying this bias will take time and the acknowledgement that there is a problem together with the willingness to do something about it. In 2020, I have seen that there has been a big movement to redress the imbalance in science at all levels. I hope that this will continue into the future so that at least some of the biases in peer review will fall away.

26.4   All reviews are not equal

If you are an editor and you receive three reviews from three researchers each suggesting something different, I have argued (in Chapter 18) that the editor should make their own decision on what action to take. But what if one of the reviewers is very negative and is a leader in their field? Should their review count equally with the others? Should their opinion be given more weight than the others? Of course, they could be using their position to influence their field, to make sure that opinions they hold are reinforced. Lee et al. (2013) provide a good overview of the potential way in which influential reviewers could bias the peer review system. But the power sits with the editor to make this decision. Interestingly, Thurner and Hanel (2011) make the point using an agent based model (much as you might use in Biological Sciences) to show that only a small number of biased (for whatever reason) reviewers are needed to seriously degrade the quality of peer review, and thus the science system as a whole.

The truth is that all reviews are not equal because some reviewers will put in more effort than others. Some will know the literature better. Some will be experts in the field that should be better placed to comment. These people are actually more likely to be less senior, PhD students, post docs or early career researchers. However, the importance for the editor is not to take account of the names of these people, their rank, their institution, or other demographics such as their gender, race or nationality. There are great editors out there who can do this, but my impression is that the majority fail. In this case, the only way to do this is by the triple blind method. Here the editors will invite the reviewers (by name) but the reviews that result will not be marked with the reviewers' names. This will make forgetting who they are easier, especially for busy editors. This would not stop these same reviews being openly published with the manuscript on completion of peer review.

26.5   Decisions rest with editors

A good editor will look at the reasoning in the reviews and make a decision in an unbiased way. A poor editor may be swayed by the perceived influence of an important reviewer irrespective of their argument. An increasing trend that I've noticed is that editors will simply take a decision that follows the consensus of all reviewers: that is, they rate all reviewers equally (see also Rothwell and Martyn, 2000). However, I would argue that this is also bad editing. Irrespective of the bias from reviewers, guarding the integrity of the process of peer review lies with editors.

Today, editors are so busy with the other duties in their jobs as academics that their decisions are hurried and expecting them to take the time and space to overcome their personal biases might be a lot to ask. Instead, I think that it is time for the Open Evaluation (OE) concept to move into the mainstream so that everyone can see how the editors came by their decision, and were not led by potential biases of their reviewers, and instead be swayed by the quality of the review and their own reading of the manuscript. This is especially important for rejected manuscripts, which is why we need the effort of this peer review recorded on preprint sites.

Another important problem with peer review comes when editors are not independent of authors. This can happen when an editor is known well by the authors. They could be in the same department or even in the same research group. Similarly, there could be a group of editors for different journals that have some *quid pro quo* arrangement, that might even be unstated, whereby their manuscripts do not undergo equal scrutiny to other manuscripts that are submitted. One could argue that whenever editors know the names of the authors, there is a conflict of interest that should be declared or risk the possibility for the system to be corrupted.

Despite all of the problems with peer review that are acknowledged above, we stick with it as the majority system in science. It could be that peer review favours exactly the same people who uphold the system and prevent it from moving into something more transparent, equal, just and fair. These are the gatekeepers, editors and reviewers who have, for the most part, managed to make their careers inside the system, and have therefore mastered it to some degree.

To you, dear reader, I can only suggest that you be aware of all the potential pitfalls with peer review, and never stop striving for something better.

26.6   The social side of peer review

There is so much more to peer review than the review. Being selected by an editor to review a manuscript represents an important standing amongst your peers. Literally it means that your opinion is valued. But there's much more to it. Doing a good job at peer review means that you improve other people's work. This help can be valued to the point where those colleagues get in touch and want to work with you. That this can happen has now been shown in a study, and has been termed the 'invisible hand' of peer review.

26.6.1   The 'invisible hand' of peer review

Dondio et al. (2019) found that reviewers were more likely to provide positive review comments to authors who were close (less than or equal to three steps) to their collaborative networks (see Adams, 2012). In this case, a close reviewer to the author was calculated by a social network where a distance of one meant that they had co-authored together (one step), co-authors of the reviewer may have collaborated with these authors (two steps), or co-authors of reviewers and authors had collaborated (three steps). Surprisingly, they obtained this result even though the journal practised a strict double-blind review system (reviewers didn't know who the authors were, and vice versa). Referees that were not close (i.e. greater than or equal to four steps) were more likely to provide more negative review comments. Those who helped authors more during peer review (i.e. asked for major revisions), were more likely to cite the manuscript, once published, and eventually more likely, than random, to publish with those same authors, even if manuscripts were eventually rejected. The authors concluded therefore that peer review may accelerate the potential for collaboration in science (Dondio et al., 2019).

This finding appears to be based on the fact that peer review can and should be constructive. Authors and peer reviewers are in fact collaborating to improve the quality of a manuscript. The process is orchestrated by an editor who can and should join in to improve the manuscript. Dondio et al. (2019) make the point that this interaction is inherently social, and the peer review therefore has a function that develops relationships within and between networks of researchers.

This evidence that peer review is a collaborative system towards the betterment of science is, to me, a sign that peer review is acting as it should. However with any social network comes the fragilities of human bias. This means that while peer review may function well for some, for others it may more often than not fail. The bigger problem is that it might depend on your sex, the colour of your skin, the name of your institution, or your country as to whether you are selected as a potential reviewer (i.e. to join the club; see Table 26.1), or having submitted your manuscript, find that peer review is going to work for you (see Davies et al., 2021). In addition, if you are never asked to review then you will never benefit from this network.

Casnici et al. (2017) tracked the fate of rejected manuscripts and showed that if the reviewers had several rounds of peer review before rejection, these manuscripts benefited later by being accepted to journals with a higher Impact Factor, and/or obtaining greater numbers of citations, even if the reviewers were instrumental in rejecting the manuscript. This suggests that in working collaboratively on a manuscript, reviewers are more likely to promote, cite and help authors. The alternative is that reviewers agree to re-review an article again because they see merit in it, even if they also see flaws. And having spent considerable effort reading the manuscript, they are more likely to remember and cite it. But this doesn't take away from the idea that reviewers and authors are collaborating in a social way.

26.7   Fixing peer review

Fixing peer review will rest with the community of biological scientists, at the level of the gatekeepers: editors and the scholarly societies that they represent. To me, it is clear that we won't fix peer review by asking our peers to be less biased, or by asking them to be more rational. We should know by now that we can't fix people in this way. For example, Khoo (2018) found that there was little improvement in reviews after reviewer training courses, even when these included feedback on previous reviews submitted. Instead, we have to plot a course for peer review whereby we accept that reviews will contain bias and irrational content, and train those in editorial positions to try to spot these, instead of manuscripts falling victim to them.

There are lots of ways by which editorial oversight can be improved. My intuition is that the crux is to find a way that makes it more efficient and objective for the editors. For example, to try to pin down reviewers on where they find fault and exactly what that fault is. There is a difference between:

- insufficient information to decide whether the experimental design was faulty and needing this clarified before a decision can be made
- finding a fundamental error in the experimental design such that the manuscript can be rejected
- insufficient power (in replicates or sampling) to reach the conclusion generated in the manuscript

A manuscript having each of these outcomes should have different fates: The first is Reject and Resubmit, the second is Reject, while the third may warrant either major/minor revisions (depending what else is problematic), or movement to another journal.

However, because peer reviewers represent a minority, this means that at times prejudices and biases will align, a more inclusive world might mean that they diverge, prompting more differences in opinions about what should happen to manuscripts. Given that it is already quite difficult to find enough reviewers, simply asking more reviewers won't fix this. Instead, we need ways by which editors can more easily come to decisions on manuscripts, taking into consideration the potential faults. This really entails journals being more transparent about what flaws in manuscripts will be considered fatal. For journals where methodological competency is all that's required (see Chapter 10 for commitment to publish), this is simple, but for many more journals (particularly those that are important for Early Career Researchers because advancement in their careers will depend on publishing there), these will be more ill-defined, editor-centric choices that are more about fashion in Biological Sciences, than good science *per se*. Removing the systematic biases is important, and something that is well worth fixing.

Hence, fixing peer review comes back to fixing problems associated with the publishing culture (and all that that entails), rather than any a simple fix-all for the myriad of existing publishing options. Preprints combined with Overlay journals offer one solution that keeps reviews with the original submission. This stops that practice of authors resubmitting their manuscripts over and over to countless journals until a pair of reviewers fail to spot a fundamental flaw. Keeping these manuscripts with their reviews on *biorXiv* (or another preprint server) represents one solution, together with another problem that good articles with biased reviews still need to overcome. I feel that this is more likely to come right with Open Publishing standards, when authors resubmit to another Overlay journal with a valid rebuttal.

Lastly, but perhaps most importantly, we have to be more realistic about the limitations of peer review. We would be better to think of peer review as a **'silver standard'** – something that some scientists agree has merit. Our problems come because our expectations of peer review are too great – a 'gold standard' it is not. Instead, we can keep the 'gold standard' for those papers that have withstood the test of time, the repeatability of the community, and acceptance into the mainstream.

27

What are predatory journals?

Predatory journals are publications that purport to be from scholarly publishing houses, but have little or no editorial oversight or peer review. They exist in order to extract the Article Processing Charge (APC) that is so ubiquitous in Open Access journals. They continue to exist because for-profit publishing is moving towards APCs, and there is little difference between what they do when compared to supposedly 'legitimate' journals. For example, some definitions of predatory journals include that their APCs far exceed their publishing costs, but this can now certainly be said of many legitimate journals (Grossmann and Brembs, 2021).

27.1 How can you tell whether or not a journal is predatory?

This is a surprisingly difficult question to answer. Predatory journals have become so sophisticated at what they do, that it can be very difficult to determine whether or not they are legitimate. Moreover, their electronically published journals can create new titles faster than the time that it takes to check that they are legitimate. An example of a publisher in the grey zone is Hindawi, once considered predatory but were later removed from Beall's list. At the time of writing, I considered that Hindawi still had some questionable practices and so suggested continuing to avoid them. However, in a new (January 2021) twist, Wiley (usually a respected publisher) acquired Hindawi for USD 298 million (Michael, 2021).

Most academics have an interaction with predatory journals through email. Indeed, the numbers of emails that academics are spammed with is astounding (VanDenBerg et al., 2021), and while the best advice is to use a spam filter, I still find that too many legitimate emails go there too. These spamming emails from predatory publishers are not straight forward and seek to manipulate the reader into submitting a manuscript (Bett, 2020). Moreover, predatory journals target the most vulnerable in the community, poorer researchers who

DOI: 10.1201/9781003220886-27

do not have English as their first language are deliberately targeted (Bett, 2020; Lund and Wang, 2020).

At the same time, legitimate journals have become increasingly predatory in their habits, and it's difficult to tell them apart from predatory journals. There was a time when it was possible to categorically state that no journal will ever approach you with a general email that invites you to contribute. However, there are now several legitimate journals that send out unsolicited emails. Realistically then, in the current publishing world, there is a continuum from predatory to legitimate. It was not always this way, and that means that as an early career researcher you are facing difficulties not faced by your mentor or other more senior academics. Not only do you need to avoid publishing in predatory journals, but you should also avoid citing their articles.

However, help is at hand. There are some definite ways in which you can determine whether you are choosing a legitimate journal. Here are my **five steps to take to safeguard your submission against a predator**.

27.1.1   How to spot a predatory journal

Use the following list in a stepwise fashion:

1. **Use an index**. Web of Science and Scopus both curate contents of legitimate journals. If your journal of choice appears in one of these, then it is very likely to be legitimate. Note that Google Scholar includes many predatory journals, so please never use this to determine whether or not a journal is legitimate. Note also that it takes a journal several years to gain enough kudos to get accepted onto Web of Science and/or Scopus. Therefore, it can still be legitimate and not be there. How to choose the right journal for your publication is covered in an earlier section (Part I). If the journal you want to publish in is not in Web of Science or Scopus, then proceed to the next step.
2. **Ask your librarian**. Librarians are fantastic sources as well as custodians of information, and journals are one of their key knowledge areas. Don't hesitate to get in touch with your librarian and ask their advice. They are likely to be very well placed to respond to your request. They may also be guardians of granting APCs at your institution, so it is in their interest to make sure that these valuable monies don't fall into the wrong hands.

3. **Ask your mentor or an experienced colleague.** It's worth doing this with them so that you can see the steps that they follow. Given that steps 1 and 2 have already come back with uncertain answers, spreading your net more widely will help with step 4. However, be warned that there are increasing numbers of senior scientists that have been caught out by predatory journals, so checking their contributors is now no cut and dry way to differentiate between them and legitimate journals.

4. **Who is on the editorial board?** Journals publish names of their editors, associate editors and the editorial board. Look through these lists and see whether there are names that you recognise. If you know any of the people, you (or your mentor) can contact and ask them about the journal (they should be happy to respond). Be warned that it is easy to place someone's name on a website, so unless they have personally told you, keep away.

5. **Check against a known list.** In the past, this might have been the first thing to do, but the number of predatory journals is proliferating so quickly that it's hard for any list to keep up. Beall's list retired in 2017. The next best list now has more than three times the number of journal names. A new list, by Simon Linacre, is sadly behind a paywall, so you can't expect to access it. One of the reasons why Beall gave up is that the new tactic for these publishers is to produce lots of new journal titles. Curating a list is real work and has implications for the publishers on it, hence you now need to pay to access an up to date list. There are more lists: Cabell's Predatory Journal Blacklist, DOAJ delisted journals, Scopus discontinued sources, etc.

27.1.2 Where's the harm in publishing with predators?

If predatory journals are becoming more like legitimate journals, where's the harm in publishing with them? Your reputation is important. As an early career researcher, your publishing record is what many people will look at first. It is all that is shown in your ORCID, Google Scholar or ResearchGate profile. It's your shop window or showroom. What prospective employers will want to see is that there are plenty of publications (appropriate for your career stage), and that they are in appropriate journals with good reputations. You might confuse having a good reputation with a high Impact Factor. The two need not be the same. High Impact Factor journals don't accept all types of submission, and you may have data that simply doesn't fit into one of their mandates. I would say that it's still important to publish, and there are many journals with good reputations where you can publish (discussion about Impact Factor is in another section).

The other reason why you would be best to avoid a predatory journal is that they attract very little in the way of scientific impact: few people will read or cite them. One thing that you definitely want for your work is for people to use it. To do this, they must read and cite it. If you publish in a predatory journal, many scientists won't even consider reading the content as it has not been, nor will it be, peer reviewed. Thus, unlike a preprint, it is not being openly offered to the community for review.

Due to the ambiguity of whether or not these papers have been peer reviewed, I would also suggest that you do not cite publications that you think may be from predatory journals. You can use the same steps (above) to determine whether or not what you want to cite is from a legitimate journal.

27.2 What to do if you have already published in a predatory journal

The first step would be to write to the publisher and withdraw the article. Whether or not you paid an APC, having it on their website is not good for your reputation. Beware, these journals don't adhere to an ethical code, and so they might refuse to withdraw your paper. Or they may want to charge an additional fee to remove it (remember that they are in it for the money).

Do not cite the paper, or put it on your CV. You can easily remove such articles from your ORCID, Google Scholar or ResearchGate profile. Don't put it in your showroom.

Prepare a statement that explains how it happened. You may not have been responsible for the submission, or aware that the publication was from a predatory publisher. However, in time you are likely to forget the exact reasons. It would be a good idea to prepare a statement, so that if you are asked (e.g. in a job interview), you can explain how it happened. People can be very understanding when provided with an explanation, but if you say that you can't remember or can't give any details, then you may sound evasive.

It's not just publishing where the predators are lurking, they are also waiting to invite you to a conference. Your work is valuable to you and to your lab, so please try to make sure that it doesn't end up in the hands of a predator!

28

Why did some journals go behind paywalls?

Academics are not (usually) superstars, nor looking for enormous numbers of readers, but there would be little point to recording our work if we had no readers, or if our work were inaccessible, and so publishing is a necessity. However, we have got into a state in which much of our work is behind a paywall, and thus inaccessible to most would be readers. Whether or not we need our work to look pretty and appealing speaks more to our readers as humans than academics. Perhaps it goes without saying that an audience is likely to be larger the more appealing the presentation, and that's not just the writing style but the layout and presentation of the text itself. And this is not new.

The first scientific journals appeared in 1665: *Journal des Sçavans*, and three months later *Philosophical Transactions of the Royal Society of London*, which is still in print today. It is clear that the papers were type set and presented in the manner of a book, perhaps analogous to a collection of short stories. At the start, these were reports of studies that were presented at meetings. Producing proceedings of learned societies became the way in which most scientific journals began. Only later did it become possible to submit a manuscript that had not been presented. And later still when publishers began to manufacture their own scholarly journals in the absence of any academic society.

Being the editor of a society journal means being elected by members of that society, and being responsible to an editorial board, normally made up of the society's members. Until very recently, and I'm thinking back to my first interactions with editors for my first few publications, submitting to the journal meant producing three (or sometimes more) double spaced hard copies of a manuscript and mailing a large and heavy envelope to the editor. Editors of bigger journals had secretaries dedicated to handling the administration of the journal. Following a telephonic enquiry, the copies were sent out to referees by post and sent back to the editorial office with a typed report often together with the marked up manuscript. Once the editor had received all reports, they communicated their decision back to the corresponding author (i.e. the one to whom correspondence was addressed) and, once accepted, the article went into production. Prior to personal computers being commonplace (only 25 years ago), each journal would have had to have had a publisher to set the type and print the pages. Clearly, this was beyond the scope of individual societies and

DOI: 10.1201/9781003220886-28

the publisher was a necessity. Libraries had to pay for copies of journals, as the cost of publishing had to be offset by the society.

The advent of desktop publishing changed the need for publishers and brought many small society journals onto a larger platform where they could produce attractive content (over the typewritten documents that had been stencil duplicated or similar) and sent around to members. However, for small societies there was no professionalism involved as it devolved to the editor to publish society material. This is where I entered the stage in 2009 when I took over as editor of the *African Journal of Herpetology.* Thankfully, email had taken the place of the postal service, but once a manuscript was accepted I was the one who needed to type-set the documents (in Quark) and send out proofs to authors (just as previous editors had done before me). Once proofs were corrected and the issue was ready, I had to find quotes from 3 printers, deliver discs and ultimately collect boxes of printed journals. Back at home, I also packed all of the copies into labelled envelopes (with some help from friends) and carried the boxes to the post office.

After the first issue, I realised that I could not do all of this work indefinitely. I knew that there were publishers who were interested in acquiring the journal into their stable (Larivière et al., 2015), and I contacted them and started negotiations. In 2011, the first copy of *African Journal of Herpetology* from a professional publisher emerged, and allowed me to go back to editing the content through peer review.

At the time, I was aware of Open Access and considered this as an option for the journal. Open Access would have required that someone pay for the type setting, and the society would still have to pay for an online dissemination platform, given that they did not have their own platform. This would have meant that authors paid for getting their manuscripts into print. And then, like today, the decision was that our authors would not be willing to pay. Other societies did opt to follow this Open Access route, with the costs being covered by the authors. For some this became an incredibly successful model, with submissions increasing as well as the Impact Factor. They demonstrate that Open Access is possible on an independent platform.

28.1 Why don't all society journals publish independently?

The first issue is that societies generate income from journals. Subscribers to print or virtual copies pay the society, and this can defray a large part of the cost of publishing otherwise carried by the members. Some make a profit, and this profit can enable the society to do more for their community of members. This could include providing small grants, subsidising conferences for students and other much appreciated initiatives. Going Open Access means losing this revenue, as well as taking on extra administrative costs.

The second issue for many societies is that their members are paying, and the councils or committees elected to represent the members do not feel that it is fair for their members to pay the additional costs of Open Access for non-members. Part of the privilege of being a member of the society is having a free (or more accurately paid through membership) copy of the society's journals. The costs are not high, and the exclusivity of members having subscription access while it is denied to others is perhaps just a hangover from the days when the only other copies were in the library. Certainly, the costs are nothing like those which authors are now charged by publishers to turn their accepted manuscripts into Open Access.

Lastly, most societies are run by a few academics who are also in jobs where they have little extra time to give. Changing the *status quo* requires additional work loads that society committee members are unwilling to take on. This is not to say that sholarly societies should not do more, they have a crucial role to play, but they will need support.

28.2   Why is there so much money in publishing science?

In the original publishing model, scholarly societies, such as The Royal Society, paid publishers to type set and print their publications. These in turn were bought by the society for their members and any libraries who subscribed to the society's content. As institutions and their libraries grew internationally, so too did the subscription base such that there was a profit to be made from the cost of the subscriptions for the paper content. Even back in those early Victorian days of scholarly publishing, publishers started their own journals (aside from any society) as they recognised their superiority in distribution (Brock, 1980). This model continued over many decades with some publishing houses growing as they acquired more journal titles from societies because there was a lot of profit to be made. The peculiarity of scholarly publishing includes the unpaid nature of authors, editors and reviewers (all of the content), and the non-equivalence of the output: that is to say that just because you have access to articles in *Nature*, they are not equivalent to those being published in *Science* – as a scientist you need to read articles from both of these publications.

Interestingly, the dawn of the internet was predicted as the downfall of the academic publisher Elsevier, because it promised the ability for academics to share their content for free (Larivière et al., 2015). Despite this, Elsevier's profit in 2012 – 13 was USD 2 billion, with a profit margin of ~40% (Larivière et al., 2015). This profit margin is so large that some have compared it favourably with street gangs selling drugs (Van Noorden, 2013; Buranyi, 2017; Logan, 2017). In the Biological Sciences, Elsevier, Springer-Nature, Wiley and Taylor-Francis control around 50% of all papers published (Larivière et al., 2015). Selling to university libraries is no longer made on print copies, but on packages of electronic journals from each of these big publishers. The deals made by individual libraries were (and are) made in strict confidence, the exact sums are unknown, but the deals made fall into the hundreds of thousands of USD for a set of publications that cover (for example) the science content of one of these publishing houses.

In 2016, it has been estimated that UK universities paid GBP ~200 million to Elsevier alone (see Logan, 2017), and global profit from science publishing was estimated at USD 9.4 billion in 2011 (Van Noorden, 2013), USD 1.1 billion for Elsevier alone (Fuchs and Sandoval, 2013).

The penalty for not subscribing is that your researchers reach a paywall when they try to access a particular paper. You will find, as I have, the luxury of visiting a very wealthy institution and having access to just about every journal title you can think of. If you are not at one of these elite institutions, then you will face a demand for money when you try to access a title that your institution does not subscribe to.

The cost of accessing a single article comes at between 25 and 50 USD (Hagve, 2020). Any members of the public who wish to read the content must pay to access it, even though these may be the same tax payers that have paid for the work to be conducted, written and peer reviewed. This is why these publisher paywalls have been branded by some as 'unethical' (e.g. Logan, 2017).

In 2014, universities in Germany abandoned all subscriptions of journals by the Dutch publishing house Elsevier, as they couldn't keep up with the 30% price increase over the previous five years, making the average cost USD 4700 per journal per year (Vogel, 2014). Despite this, Elsevier continued to allow these universities access to their content for free, before negotiating another (secret) more amenable deal to them. Somehow the publishers had managed to turn the ease of distribution of articles over the internet to their advantage, via effective paywalls.

Open Access titles came about in the early 2000s as the need for hard printed copies fell away and academics became comfortable handling all of their publications as pdfs. In the Biological Sciences, *PLOS ONE* was the title that revolutionised the market, quickly becoming the single biggest journal. What caught the eyes of the publishers was the article processing charge (APC) that academics seemed to be prepared to pay. When they first started, *PLOS ONE* cost USD ~1300 for its APC (Khoo, 2019). Publishers quickly started titles with similar no Impact Factor goals. Competitive titles began at the same cost as *PLOS ONE*, but once these titles became established, with higher Impact Factors, they quickly increased their APC (Khoo, 2019). Publishers are adept at pricing their titles at what libraries and authors are prepared to pay, such that for-profit publications are regularly more expensive than non-profit journals (Björk & Solomon, 2015). Between 2012 and 2018, the increase in APCs from several Gold OA publishers grew at between 2.6 and 6 times the rate of inflation (Khoo, 2019). In their analyses of drivers of APC for OA journals, Budzinski et al. (2020) found several variables that explained the vast difference in APCs of different journals. Impact Factor played an important role, but so too did market power of the publishers (presumably the ability to distribute the title and content), the hybrid model (Gold OA or Hybrid OA), and the concentration of disciplines that they cover.

Librarians analysed content that was Open Access finding that it was more highly cited, and so academics began to look for the potential to publish Open Access. The publishers were happy to oblige, and in the early days conducted 'double dipping' charging both the APC for the authors, and collecting full revenue for subscription to hybrid journals by universities (Pinfield et al., 2016). It was only in May 2018 that Knowledge Unlatched formed an alliance to prevent double-dipping in Open Access publications.

The end to double-dipping, now mandated by governments (Pinfield et al., 2016), has led to even more complicated publishing deals known as **transformative publisher agreements** (Table 28.1). These deals are said to lead to even greater profits for the publishers (Poynder, 2020). With these agreements, researchers from universities that have full subscriptions to certain publishers will receive free Gold OA for any journals in the package and their authors will be able to publish OA inside the same publisher's journals. In effect, the price of the OA is offset against the cost of the subscription. As you may have noticed, this could quickly start a bias in the publishing trends of academics from some (middle income) institutions publishing with certain titles, because they receive the benefit of OA. Those from privileged institutions will continue to publish anywhere they can, and the real losers will be those from poorer institutions and especially middle-income countries, who cannot afford transformative agreements, and cannot afford to provide their researchers with costs to cover APCs (Measey, 2018). For these researchers, there will be a reduced set of journals that they can submit manuscripts to. This is the current reality that increasing numbers of researchers find themselves in.

On the face of it, Plan S makes total sense (Schiltz, 2018). If all papers published by European researchers are Open Access, then everyone can read them and there is no more need for paywalls. Unfortunately, the way in which Plan S has been implemented has only been for wealthy European institutions. Others are left to continue to pay a hefty APC price for OA publishing, and their libraries pay a subscription to access journal content (Hagve, 2020). There is a real possibility that the USA and China will take other routes to OA, causing a schism in publishing, more complex agreements and even more profits for publishers (Poynder, 2020).

TABLE 28.1: How publishers make a profit. There are many ways in which publishers can generate income from publishing scientific journals.

Funding source	From society journals	From their own journals	From Open Access	From copyright
Old subscription model (mostly obsolete)	X	X	-	-
Selling bundles to university libraries (undisclosed sums – millions of USD)	X	X	-	-
Selling articles of large back catalogues (~10% goes to society)	X	X	-	-
Article Process Charging	-	-	X	-
Double dipping	X	X	-	-
Transformative publisher agreements	X	X	X	-
Copyright content	X	X	-	X

Another way that publishers make money is through copyright on the content of their very large back catalogues. There are a lot of text books written for undergraduate students, and this is a large profit making publishing model in and of itself. When you look at the examples given in text books, they are often taken directly from peer reviewed papers. The publishers of the text book will pay for the content that they get from the pages of journals where they are under copyright. This can be very lucrative for the publishers who retain copyright from the authors. The advent of Creative Commons licensing has meant that it is now very easy to make the content of journals available for anyone to use. Happily, most Open Access journals have taken this route.

28.2.1 How could such a profitable business lead to making a loss?

To be fair, we should also consider that some publishers have not (always) been able to turn a profit, even when their turnover is in millions of USD. One such beleaguered publisher is PLOS. Despite growing exponentially in the early noughties, becoming the world's biggest academic publisher in 2013,

PLOS has not managed to turn a profit since 2015 (Davies, 2019). At the time of writing (May 2021), the APC on a *PLOS ONE* article was USD 1749, while other PLOS titles ranged from USD 2100 to 4000. This begs the question, how much does it cost to process an article? Data from the PLOS Financial Overview suggests that processing your article costs USD ~315, with another USD ~262 to keep it online.

So where does the rest of the money go? PLOS spend the bulk of your APCs on the editorial aspects of publishing. Remember that PLOS don't pay academic editors, but they do have huge financial burdens of the salaries of their own editorial staff. PLOS is based in San Francisco, California, which just happens to be one of the most expensive cities in the world to live in. Chief among their many options are to raise the costs of your APCs in order to pay their staff, or move their operation to somewhere cheaper. Interestingly, two of the other large OA outfits, MDPI and Frontiers, are both based in Switzerland, one of the most expensive countries in the world in which to pay salaried staff.

Most recently, PLOS announced a new funding model to keep themselves afloat that spreads the cost of their APC among the authors and aims to cap profits at 10% (Else, 2021). The new scheme, Community Action Publishing, sees a return to the institutional subscription model where institutions will be charged proportionately at the rate their academics publish in PLOS. Great if your institutions can afford to opt in. If not, you can expect to face your proportion of the APC now as a co-author (instead of only the corresponding author paying).

Time will tell whether PLOS can make their new financial model work in order to keep their staff in the comfort to which they have become accustomed. No doubt we will see more of these new funding models as the increasingly bloated OA market attempts to consolidate itself, while still feeding on the funds of the global tax payer.

In case you hadn't realised, there is no advertising (at least in Biological Sciences – some medical journals do have advertising). You do see adverts when you are browsing the content of *Nature* and *Science*. Oddly, this doesn't make them any cheaper to publish in, but presumably does increase the profits for their publishers. In the last 10 years, big publishers have shifted their strategy from making money on publishing towards collecting and selling data (Posada and Chen, 2018; Brembs et al., 2021; Pooley, 2021). Their strategy appears to be buying up the tools that academics use in a workflow including: discovery, analysis, writing, publication, outreach and assessment. Once this entire workflow is captured, the publishers can track individual users across it and sell this information to the institutions that employ them (Posada and Chen, 2018; Christl, 2021), or third parties that may profit from knowing what you read and write (Pooley, 2021). All of this is reminiscent of the Cambridge Analytica scandal which is alleged to have manipulated election results in the UK and USA in 2016. If we want academia to be captured, we can continue to keep our eyes on the highest Impact Factors.

28.3   What will it take to break the vicious cycle?

We need new models for publishing. Society journals are still kings in this game and ultimately hold the cards for moving away from stoking the profits of publishing companies. What we have seen in recent years is that journals can come from nowhere to become dominant players in the system. Think *PLOS ONE*, and the even more recent meteoric rise of *Scientific Reports*. These mega Open Access journals didn't exist ten years ago. And they don't need to exist ten years from now. What is needed is for the actual costs of publishing (not those currently inflated by publishers - see Grossmann and Brembs, 2021) to be covered by the institutions that employ the academics. This could cover typesetting (fulfilling our irrational desire for 'fancy layouts') and the additional IT infrastructure (on-line submission system and online dissemination platform). Most (if not all) societies are not-for-profit organisations, and only need to cover the costs of publishing.

28.3.1   A role for scholarly societies and libraries

Scholarly societies have an important role to play in leading change in the scientific publishing model. Not only do societies organise their own membership, and elect members to positions, but they have the potential to make sure that there is equity in their executive committees. Indeed, previous studies have shown that women leaders promote more equitable societies, but globally most societies in the Biological Sciences are still dominated by men (Potvin et al., 2018). Promoting equity and representation of a society's membership is an important step on the road to transparency, and to make the shift from closed to open science. Societies need to be led by the desire of their members for Diamond Open Access society journals, now that it has been established that this is possible through overlay journals.

Without publishers, we still need to organise academics at a level beyond the individual and spanning institutions. This means elevating the importance of scholarly societies (Harington, 2020), with all of the additional benefits that these bring (e.g. networking, conference organisation, newsletters, socialising, mentoring, stewardship, community of practice, ethics, outreach, etc.). However, far from relying on the publishers being the sources of income for societies (Harington, 2020), we need a professional society model (such as is seen in medicine and other vocationally orientated disciplines) whereby the relationship between academics and their societies is strengthened through their institutions.

28.4   Can we afford not to change?

If you are from a rich country or institution, then you can probably afford the current system. Those who cannot are researchers in middle-income countries and disadvantaged institutions. In some cases, the cost of publishing Open Access is greater than the cost of the research. These are insurmountable costs for many researchers. We have a massive hole in scientific contributions from the poorest of nations, and the current Open Access models will see their work being the most hidden from view, while the countries paying for their work do so disproportionately. But even middle-income countries could be winners in a new Open Access model. By sourcing the relevant IT skills in the country, governments of middle-income countries could facilitate the content of their own society's with relative comfort.

28.5   Societies need money. Editors can't be publishers.

We desperately need good, free editorial management software. There are some free versions out there, but what we need are open source versions that are at least as good, if not better, than existing platforms (e.g. ScholarOne; Editorial Manager). Galipeau et al. (2016) make the point about the ever expanding role of editors in the modern publishing era. There is no scope for editors to take on extra work.

We need an Open LaTeX interface with robust templates for all societal journals. Ideally, this would be packaged with the above editorial management software. This must have the ability to cope with figures and equations, and the unusual demands that some society journals have.

We need a solution for hosting and disseminating the Open Access society journals (and their supplementary information if not hosted elsewhere) in perpetuity. This last point is perhaps the most expensive, and almost certainly requires government assistance. Maybe this is an interesting use of the block-chain with libraries keeping the data. It would be an interesting way to build a digital object identifier (DOI) with editor and referee unique IDs, and the document's information hanging off.

We need to take back our content stuck behind paywalls. Yes, it's time for you all to dig up those old submitted manuscripts and submit them to an institutional repository where they can be accessed for free.

28.6 A paywall is never acceptable wherever you put it

Any paywall, whether it be high (e.g. EUR 9500 for *Nature* in 2020), or considerably lower (e.g. EUR 900 for *NeoBiota* in 2020), is a wall that excludes many researchers, and certainly those from many middle-income countries. While previously I called for the source of these publishing fees to become public (Measey, 2018), which I suggest would show that for a great majority of researchers, publishing fees are coming from research funds. Now I think that our energies would be better spent removing all paywalls: Diamond Open Access for everyone.

If current trends continue, scientists from low-income countries will be granted full fee waivers. Many journals use the Hinari Eligibility list of countries[1] to separate Group A (free access) and Group B (low cost access – normally billed at a 50% reduction in fees). The lists are made up from five global economic and development criteria. Middle-income countries are missing from these lists, and receive no support for fee waivers. Their governments provide scientists with no means of paying fees. Scientists who pay fees often do so from their own research budgets. The increasing number of journals that charge unjustifiably high publishing costs are forcing middle-income countries' scientists away from Open Access journals.

Until we have Diamond Open Access for all, having the paywall after publication is the preferable reality for most researchers, as most of us cannot afford to pay anything as they simply don't have this type of discretionary funds. They do have to publish our work, and would rather that it was out there behind a paywall, than not out there at all. Placing the paywall before publication simply stops many from publishing. In the words of Peterson et al. (2019), "do not replace one problem with another." We are all quick and ready to agree that Open Access is the best way forward for all scientific results, so this means Diamond Open Access for everyone.

28.7 The answer lies inside our university libraries

University libraries have undergone a massive transformation over the last 20 years. During my PhD, I made a weekly visit to the library to physically pick up the latest issues of all the journals that came through the postal service from all over the world. Librarians arranged these issues on the shelves and

[1] http://www.who.int/hinari/eligibility/en/

eventually sent them off for binding into volumes and then worried about the physical space that was available inside the library as every year publication inflation (Larivière and Costas, 2016) meant more pages to be supported within their walls.

For papers that I found out about but were not in the library, I had a stack of postcards that were specifically for reprint requests, and I enthusiastically filled them out and posted them off to researchers the world over. The post held a weekly haul of fat envelopes filled with offprints that were frequently more than I'd asked for. Many researchers would sign the top with personal messages – halcyon days perhaps. But there are better days ahead.

Like others, I think that the logical solution to our problem with publishers is to turn to our university libraries to curate our academic outputs (Fang and Casadevall, 2012). There are clear reasons why it makes sense for libraries to take on the roll as publishers. Most of us are employed by universities or research institutions that also fund libraries. Linking the work we do (writing, reviewing and editing) more closely with our institutions would result in a greater appreciation for this part of our workload. Libraries have fantastic networks, and are our professional long-term storage partners. They developed efficient and impressive information technology (IT) long before it hit most academic departments. Their inter-library networks are what we now need to disseminate the knowledge that we generate without any walls. The idea of libraries as the new publishers isn't new. Raju and Pietersen (2017) proposed this as a solution in Africa. Here I extend the same idea as a practical way of publishing academic journals for the world.

To help the budget of your university library, you can introduce them to **Unsub** (unsub.org). This software helps librarians evaluate usage of journals in their subscriptions, and helps them understand their cancellation options. When libraries spend less on subscriptions, they'll have more money to kick start Open Access publishing.

28.8   Do we need a fancy layout?

Once the storage and dissemination of our contributions are taken care of, the only service left from the publishers is a fancy layout. This is mostly a historical legacy. I have to admit that I really like seeing my work being nicely produced and printed. But I'm happy to give this up if it means demolishing paywalls. In reality, LaTeX can solve most of these problems so that we simply use the journal (library) produced template, that will need minimal manipulation afterwards. I feel sure that those who are hung up on the importance of their layout can find students at their own institutions who will be happy to provide layout services for a reasonable fee. No doubt, there will be some institutions that will invest extra to have nicer layouts for their journals. But I feel confident that this will not change the impact, or any other journal metrics, as academics will value the papers for what they contain rather than what they look like. Nothing about the contents of the highest ranking journals suggests that Impact Factor is consistently related to research quality.

If our futures lie with the overlay model of publishing, then I suggest that we need to have less reliance on international storage of (what are currently) 'preprints', and instead a closer relationship between university libraries and scholarly societies is needed for preprint storage. If you have read this far, then I hope that you will join the call for Diamond Open Access – no paywalls for anyone.

28.9   Giving up the obsession with metrics

Another key move will be having all academic institutions and funders adopting the San Francisco Declaration on Research Assessment (known as DORA) in order to stop hiring staff based on their publishing metrics, and the negative impacts that this is known to have (Casadevall and Fang, 2012). This will have an impact on many aspects of science including the current way in which science is funded on a 'winner takes all' basis (Casadevall and Fang, 2012). Many suggestions for reforming science are out there, but when the participants are still ruled by the cult of metrics, it is hard to imagine the necessary reforms taking place (Fang and Casadevall, 2012).

29

Are researchers writing more, and is more better?

The idiom 'publish or perish' suggests that researchers will increase their output in order to obtain positions and promotions. And if a researcher's productivity is measured by their publication output, shouldn't we all be writing more papers? Certainly, it appears that more papers are being published (see Figure 29.1). An estimate for the total number of scholarly articles in existence was 50 million in 2009, with more than half of these published in the years from 1984 (Jinha, 2010).

Similarly, if we are all be writing more, then wouldn't some people start publishing two (or more) papers, when one would be adequate? This idea of 'salami slicing' to inflate outputs would be an understandable strategy if researchers were all trying to increase their output. Alternatively, the names of authors might be added to papers in which they did not make significant input via ghost authorship or hyperauthorship (see Cronin, 2001, for an interesting historical perspective, and Part I).

A study by Fanelli and Larivière (2016) has a new take on the above questions, by asking whether researchers are actually writing more papers now than they did 100 years ago. They used the Web of Science to look for unique authors (more than half a million of them) and determine whether the first year of publication and the total number of publications resulted in an increasing trend. Fanelli and Larivière's (2016) trend line for biology is very stable at around 5.5 publications whether you started publishing in 1900 or 2000 (note that earth science and chemistry do both increase dramatically).

But it is possible that these figures could be explained by the fact that the culture in publishing in Biological Sciences has changed a great deal since 1900. One hundred years ago, it was very unlikely that any postgraduate students would publish articles in peer reviewed journals. Moreover, it was also acceptable for advisers to take the thesis work of their students and write it up in monographs. This has certainly changed with the ranks of authors now being swelled considerably so that many more authors are likely to be included on only a single publication in which they participated (see Measey, 2011). I interpret this as the Biological Sciences becoming more democratic, with more of the people that contribute to the work receiving the credit.

DOI: 10.1201/9781003220886-29

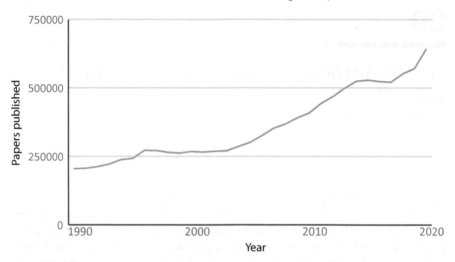

FIGURE 29.1: The growth in the number of papers published in Life Sciences over time. The number of papers published. Data from www.scopus.com.

29.0.1   At what rate is the literature increasing?

Using several databases (Web of Science, Scopus, Dimensions and Microsoft Academic) back to the beginning of their collections at the start of scientific journals in the mid 1600s, Bornmann et al. (2020) calculated the inflation rate of scientific literature to run at 4.02%, such that the literature will double in 16.8 years (Bornmann et al., 2020). This means that there is literally twice as much published by 2020 as there was in 2003.

Although the early period of scientific publishing was notably slower than today, it is since the mid-1940s (following the end of 'World War II') that science has seen an exponential growth in productivity, with annual growth of 5.1%, and a doubling time of 13.8 years (Bornmann et al., 2020).

29.0.2   If more is being published, will Impact Factors increase?

Yes, there is inflation of Impact Factors. If the numbers of citations per paper remains constant, then the Impact Factor of journals should increase annually at 5%. My impression (see Measey, 2011) is that citations are increasing in papers as the literature increases, which suggests that Impact Factor will grow at a faster rate.

29.1 Are some authors unfeasibly prolific?

How many articles could you publish in a year before you could be described as 'unfeasibly prolific'? This question was posed in a study that examined prolific authors in four fields of medicine (Wager et al., 2015). This publication piqued my interest as it turns out that the authors decided that researchers with more than 25 publications in a year were unfeasibly prolific, as this would be the equivalent of '>1 publication per 10 working days'. Their angle was to suggest that publication fraud was likely, and that funders should be more circumspect when accepting researchers productivity as a metric. Looking back through the peer review of this article (which is a great aspect of many *PeerJ* articles), I'm astounded that only one reviewer questioned the premise that it's infeasible to author that number of papers in a year.

I have published >25 papers and book chapters in a year, and I know other people who do this regularly. To me, there is no question that (a) it is possible and (b) that they really are the authors – with no question of fraud. Firstly, the idea that prolific authors constrain their activity to 'working days' is naïve. Most will be working throughout a normal weekend, and working in the early morning and late evening, especially in China (see Barnett et al., 2019). A hallmark of a prolific author would be emails early in the morning and/or late at night. This gives you an indication of their working hours, and how they are struggling to keep up with correspondence on top of writing papers.

Authorship of a publication is often the result of several years of work, and it can be at many different levels of investment (see Part 1). Thus, from my perspective, when I look at authoring a lot of publications it reflects the activity of the initial concept for the work, raising of money, conducting the field work or experiment, analysing the data and then writing it up (with the subsequent submission and peer review time – see Part I). Often, the work conducted by students who lead the publications, many years later, are the culmination of many years of investment of both time and money. And in the Biological Sciences, good study systems keep giving.

29.2 Salami-slicing

'Salami-slicing' is different things to different people. While many people refer to salami-slicing as the multiplication of papers into as many papers as possible, or slicing research into 'least publishable units', others are referring to publishing the same paper more than once in different journals. In the latter case, this should be considered self-plagiarism at best and fraud at worst. If you find examples of dual publications, these should result in retractions. Instances don't need to be exact copies. I edited a submission where one of the referees alerted me to the fact that the same data with a very similar question had already been published two years previously. In this instance, I passed the submission to the ethical panel of the journal who rejected it, and flagged the authors for scrutiny in the case of future submissions. Note that instances where conference abstracts are printed in a journal does not prevent you from publishing a full paper of this work. I would maintain, however, that you should rewrite the abstract to prevent self-plagiarism (Hall et al., 2021; Measey, 2021).

During the production of any dataset, you are likely to find that you are able to answer more questions than you originally set out to ask when you first proposed the research (i.e. preregistration; see Part I). The question you will be left with is: whether you should be adding these *post hoc* questions (questions that arise after the study) to the manuscripts that you planned to write when you proposed the research, or whether these should be published as separate publications – clearly identified as *post hoc* questions? The realities of publishing in scientific journals means that in many instances you will be restricted by the number of words a journal will accept. This will mean that for certain outputs it will not be possible for you to ask additional *post hoc* questions, or potentially all the questions you wanted to report in the preregistered plan.

There is nothing wrong with writing papers based purely on findings that you came across during the study: *post hoc* questions. There is a clear role in scientific publishing of natural history observations. But that any publication (or part of a publication) that results must indicate that it results from a *post hoc* study. To my way of thinking, it would be more useful if journals had separate sections for such studies, with other publications only stemming from from those that can show a preregistered plan. This would clearly improve transparency in publishing, and avoid accusations of p-hacking or HARKing.

Although 'salami-slicing' is the preoccupation of many authors and gatekeepers, there is evidence that more experimental data and analyses are now required to meet the standards of modern publishing (in some journals) compared to 30 years ago (Vale, 2015). As we move towards a more open and equitable way of sharing our data, we should see an increase the the total amount of evidence that can be put towards answering more questions. However, metric based assessments will always tempt some individuals to game the system (Chapman et al., 2019), resulting in a need to be aware of potential 'salami-slicing'. At what point does the separation of research questions into different papers become 'salami slicing'? There is no simple answer to this question, and editors are likely to disagree (Tolsgaard et al., 2019). However, there are ways in which you as an author can make sure that your work is transparent, and therefore that you are not accused of 'salami slicing'. First is the preregistration of your research plan. Second is to preprint any unpublished papers that are referenced in your submission. There are also guidelines from COPE on the: 'Systematic manipulation of the publication process' (COPE, 2018b). And the last is to be transparent when you publish *post hoc* research.

In manuscripts where another very similar study is cited by the authors, but not available to reviewers or editors, there should be a 'salami slicing' red flag. Obviously, when you produce a number of outputs from a research project, they are likely to be linked and therefore cited by each other. However, when these are not available to reviewers and editors (as preprints or as preregistration of the questions), authors should expect to be asked for these manuscripts to demonstrate that they are not salami-slicing. Perhaps worse, however, is when authors deliberately hide any citation to another very similar work. In the end, we have to rely on the integrity of the researchers not to be unethical or dishonest.

29.3   Is writing a lot of papers a good strategy?

This is a question of long standing, and one that you may find yourself asking at some point early on in your career. I'd suggest that the answer will be more about the sort of person that you are, or the lab culture you experience, over any strategy that you might consciously decide. If you tend towards perfectionism, this will likely result in fewer papers that (I hope) you'd consider to be of high quality. If on the other hand your desire were to finish projects and move on, you'd be more likely to tend towards more papers. It is clear that the current climate leads towards the latter strategy, with increasing numbers of early career researchers bewildered at the idea of increasing their publication metrics (Helmer et al., 2020). But what should you do?

Given that the 'best' personality type lies somewhere in the middle, you can decide for yourself whether you identify with one side more than the other. But which is the better strategy? Vincent Larivière and Rodrigo Costas (2016) tried to answer this question by considering how many papers unique authors wrote and seeing how this relates to their share of authoring a paper in the top 1% of cited papers. Their result showed clearly that for researchers in the life sciences, writing a lot of papers was a good strategy if you started back in the 1980s. However, for those starting after 2009, the trend was reversed with those authors writing more papers less likely to have a 'smash hit' paper (in the top 1% of cited papers). Maybe the time scale was too short to know. After all, if you started publishing in 2009 and had >20 papers by 2013 then you have been incredibly (but not unfeasibly) prolific. Other studies continue to show that in the life sciences, writing more papers still provides returns towards having papers highly cited: the more papers you author, the higher the chance of having a highly cited paper (Sandström and van den Besselaar, 2016).

One aspect not considered by Larivière and Costas (2016) is that becoming known as a researcher who finishes work (resulting in a publication) is likely to make you more attractive to collaborators. Thus, publishing work is likely to get you invited to participate in more work. Obviously, quality plays a part in invitations to collaborative work too. Thus pulling the argument back to the centre ground. However, many faculty in North America (and particularly female faculty) seem to believe that writing more papers is considered desirable for review, promotion and tenure, including a greater number of publications per year (Niles et al., 2020). Whether or not this is the case within their institutions, that faculty consider it desirable may be part of the trend to publish more.

There are other scenarios in which you might be encouraged to write more. In Denmark, for example, research funding is apportioned to universities based on the number of outputs their researchers generated in a point system, where higher ranked journals get more points. This resulted in researchers in the life sciences changing their publication strategy with a notable increase in publications in the highest points bracket following this change (Deutz et al., 2021).

You may find yourself becoming preoccupied about which is the best strategy for you, not because you want to, but because your institution is relying on you to pull your weight in their assessment exercise. University rankings are now very important, and big universities like to be ranked highly for research, which depends (in part) on the quantity and quality of their output.

29.3.1   Natural selection of bad science

In 2016, Smaldino and McElreath proposed that ever increasing numbers of publications not only leads to bad science, but is currently selected for in an academic environment where publishing is considered as a currency. They argued that the most productive laboratories will be rewarded with more grant funding, larger numbers of students, and that these students will learn about the methods and benefits of prolific publication. When these 'offspring' of the prolific lab look for jobs, they are more likely to be successful as they have more publications themselves. An academic environment that rewards increasing numbers of publications eventually selects towards methodologies that produce the greatest number of publishable results. To show that this leads to a culture of 'bad science', Smaldino and McElreath (2016) conducted an analysis in trends over time of statistical power in behavioural science publications.

Over time, better science should be shown by researchers increasing their statistical power as this will provide studies with lower error rates. However, increasing the statistical power of experiments takes more time and resources, resulting in fewer publications. Their results, from review papers in social and behavioural sciences, suggested that between 1960 and 2011 there had been no trend towards increasing statistical power. Biological systems, whether they be academics in a department or grass growing in experimental pots, will respond to the rewards generated in that system. When grant funding bodies and academic institutions reward publishing as a behaviour, it is inevitable that the behaviour of researchers inside that system will respond by increasing their publication output. Moreover, if those institutions maintain increasing numbers of researchers in temporary positions, those individuals are further incentivised to become more productive to justify their continued contracts, or the possibility of obtaining a (more permanent) position elsewhere. Eventually, this negative feedback, or gamification of publishing metrics, produces a dystopian and dysfunctional academic reality (Helmer et al., 2020).

An example of this kind of confirmation bias driven publishing effect towards bad science can be found in the literature of fluctuating asymmetry, and in particular those studies on human faces (Van Dongen, 2011). Back in the 1990s, there was a flurry of high profile articles purporting preference for symmetry (and against asymmetry) in human faces. The studies were (relatively) cheap and fast to conduct as the researchers had access to hundreds of students right on their doorsteps. The studies not only hit the top journals, but were very popular in the mainstream media as scientists were apparently able to predict which faces were most attractive.

Stefan van Dongen (2011) hypothesised that if publication bias was leading to bad science in studies of fluctuating asymmetry in human faces, there would be a negative association between effect size and sample size. However, effect sizes can also be expected to be smaller in larger studies as these may come with less accurate measurements (see Jennions and Møller, 2002). This negative association should not change depending on the stated focus of the study; i.e. if the result was the primary or secondary outcome. However, van Dongen found that in studies where the relationship between fluctuating asymmetry and attractiveness was a secondary outcome (not the primary focus of the study), the overall effect size did not differ from zero and no association between effect size and sample size was found. This was in contrast to the studies where the fluctuating asymmetry-attractiveness was a primary focus, suggesting that there was important publication bias in this area of research.

Where others have looked, publication bias has been found and is particularly associated with a decreasing effect size that correlates with journal Impact Factor: i.e. once the large effect is published in a big journal, the natural selection of bad science results in publication bias, and diminishing effect sizes that ripple through lower Impact Factor journals (Munafò et al., 2007; Brembs et al., 2013; Smaldino and McElreath, 2016), while negative results disappear almost entirely (Fanelli, 2012). One can presume that negative results exist, but their authors either do not bother to write up the results, or that journals won't publish them.

29.3.2   Does all of this tell us that publishing more is bad?

Although I would agree that continuing the exponential trend in numbers of publications is unsustainable, more publications are not bad *per se*. Instead, we need to be more careful about what we do and don't publish, as well as the reasons why we publish. As long as we are conducting science and communicating our results, there should be no problem. Our problems arrive with publication bias, especially not publishing negative results (Nissen et al., 2016) and chasing ever higher Impact Factors. The direct result of a system driven by Impact Factor and author publication metrics is that we will have a generation of scientists at the top institutions that are trained not to conduct the best science, but to generate publications that can be sold to the best journals. We should be deeply suspicious of any claim of linkage between top journals and quality (Brembs et al., 2013). Indeed, what we see increasingly is that the potential rewards of publishing in top Impact Factor journals leads not only to bad science, but increasingly to deliberate fraud. Continuing along this path threatens to undermine the entire scientific project[1], and places science and scientists as just another stakeholder in a system ruled by economic markets, and their promotion of the fashion of the day (Brembs et al., 2013; Casadevall and Fang, 2012).

---

[1] howtowriteaphd.com/lifescientific.html

30

When should you correct or retract your paper?

Once your Version of Record is published, any changes that you may wish to make will result in a separate correction publication. In extreme cases, you may even need to retract the paper. The different options available in many journals to correct your paper are shown in Table 30.1. If you are in doubt about exactly what kind of correction you need, read the guidelines from the Council of Science Editors (www.councilscienceeditors.org) and the Committee on Publication Ethics (publicationethics.org) (COPE) (Barbour et al., 2009).

TABLE 30.1: Journals have a number of different ways in which to correct the published Version of Record. You may not need a full retraction to set your study straight. Source: Council of Science Editors.

Action	Example	Conclusions impacted	Issued by
Corrigendum/ erratum/ correction	Important typos/incorrect figure legends or tables/author name or address issues	Not	Author
Expression of concern	Data appear unreliable/misconduct suspected	Undetermined	Editor (perhaps through information received)
Partial retraction	One aspect of the study is corrupted/Inappropriate analysis	Overall findings remain	Author or Editor
Full retraction	Majority of the study is corrupted/Evidence of misconduct/Work is invalidated	Yes	Author or Editor

DOI: 10.1201/9781003220886-30

30.1   Making a correction to a published paper

It is very unlikely that you will be in a position where you will need to think about retracting your paper. If you notice a mistake, especially one that results in a difference to how the results are presented, then you should approach the editor about publishing a correction (also termed a *corrigendum* or *erratum* – plural *errata*).

Because a *corrigendum* is a change to the VoR, it will result in what is in effect an additional separate publication (with its own DOI). This will succinctly point out the error and how this should be rectified. In the journal, this will only be a few lines. In addition, on the site of the original publication, the journal will place a notice that there has been a correction, and provide a permalink to the correction. However, it results in a lot of extra administrative work for everyone, so it's best avoided if at all possible. This is another reason why it's worth taking your time when checking your proofs.

Another way to avoid having to make a *corrigendum* is to ensure that all co-authors are happy with the original submission, the resubmission and the proofs (i.e. get it right before you submit it).

Mistakes do occur, and it is likely to be some time after the publication that you might find that there was an error. Errors such as typos, or mistakes in the introduction or discussion are unlikely to warrant a *corrigendum*. However, if the error is in the way that the results were calculated, or causes a change in the significance, then you should consider making a *corrigendum*. If you feel that it is necessary, do consult your co-authors before taking it to the editor. It is well worth having someone else check your new calculation, as the last thing you want is a compounded error.

If the mistake is systemic, and changes all of the results, their significance and/or the validity of the conclusion, then you need to consider a full retraction.

30.2   Expression of concern

An expression of concern lies between a correction and a retraction. An expression of concern can precede a retraction, but suggests that the editors are seriously worried about something being wrong with the publication. For example, a paper published in *Proceedings of the National Academy of Sciences* that used an unusual mutant strain of *Chlamydomonas* (a genus of green algae) was placed under an official 'Editorial Expression of Concern' when the editors learned that the authors would not share their strain with any other researchers (Berenbaum, 2021). Clearly, this notice could be removed if, for example, the authors agreed to share their strain and their findings were replicated. However, if they continue to refuse, the editors could also fully retract the paper.

This is an unusual case, but shows how the editors are prepared to take their journal's policy seriously, as a requirement of submission is that authors must be prepared to share any unique reagents described in their papers, or declare restrictions up front. Failure of these authors to follow through with the transparency declared on submission could mean that these authors have their paper retracted. Finding out this sort of information takes time, and so there is often a lag in the retraction window (Figure 30.1).

30.3 A retraction is unusual

A retraction of a paper is when your paper is effectively 'unpublished'. This happens at the discretion of the editor (and often the entire editorial board), and is a very serious issue. Retractions are rare. Reasons for retractions vary. It could be that a piece of equipment was later found to have malfunctioned or was calibrated incorrectly (Anon, 2018). A cell line was misidentified. Or they can be through no fault of the authors. For example, Toro et al. (2019) had their manuscript rejected by *Journal of Biosciences*, but due to an administrative error, the article was printed in an issue, and later retracted. However, the top reason for retraction is now misconduct (Fang et al., 2012; Brainard and You, 2018), and this is hardly surprising given the crazy incentives that many scientists receive to publish in journals with top Impact Factors. Another important factor with retractions is that they appear to be more common in journals with higher Impact Factors (Brembs et al., 2013), and this should not surprise us as these journals are prone to publishing studies with confirmation bias (Forstmeier et al., 2017; Measey, 2021).

Although retractions are rare in life sciences, 0.06% of all papers published between 1990 and 2020, they appear to be on the increase in the last 30 years: from around 0.5 to over 15 papers per 10,000 published (see Figure 30.1). It takes a mean time of nearly 2 years between notification of problems with a paper, and issuing a correction or retraction (Grey et al., 2021), but this belies a bimodal distribution in retraction times with the first hump coming from self-correcting authors, or clerical errors from journals coming within months of the original date of publication. The second hump is usually associated with fraud, and comes after several years of investigations by institutions often with added legal frustrations.

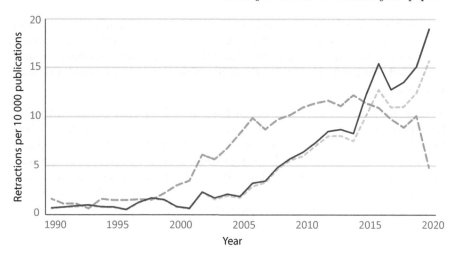

FIGURE 30.1: The growth of retractions in Life Sciences journals over time. The three lines show when the original paper is published (dashed line) and when a correction, expression of concern or retraction are made (solid black line). Articles that are finally retracted (dotted line) are only a part of those with other issues after 2008. While the number of papers published that are later retracted appears to take a turn downward from 2014, this may simply represent the lag before they are later retracted. This data came from the Retraction Watch database, selecting only data from Basic Life Sciences and Environment. The data is normalised by dividing the total number of publications (as taken from SCOPUS) in this area for the year by 10,000, and multiplying this by numbers of original or retracted papers.

Retractions showed a steep uptake in 2011, when a number of laboratories made multiple retractions (see Fang and Casadevall, 2011; Brainard and You, 2018). A single publisher was responsible for pulling a great many of the retracted papers in 2011, and this spike in retractions isn't seen in the life sciences (Oransky, 2011; Brainard and You, 2018). What is clear from Figure 30.1 is that the rising trend in retractions (black line) appears to have been unaffected by the 2011 spike in other subject areas. Claims that retractions are levelling off (Brainard and You, 2018), are not matched by the data.

30.3.1 How do you know if a paper you cited is later retracted?

Citations to retracted papers are not uncommon, and often positively cite the paper even when the retraction has been made for misconduct (Bar-Ilan and Halevi, 2017). This suggests that most authors are simply not aware of the retracted status of many publications. Of course, if you visit the publisher's website, you should see a clear notification at the Version of Record, that points to the retraction notice, but this is not always the case. In general, publishers seem very shy about their retractions, and it can be difficult to track down retractions that should be clear for everyone to see. Indeed, if publishers did their due diligence on notifications on retractions, and this were entered into CrossRef, we wouldn't need an independent database like the Retraction Watch database.

If you downloaded the article before it was retracted, then you will not be aware of what has happened unless you are following that particular publication. Similarly, if you get your search results from Google Scholar, there is no indication that a paper has been retracted. Scopus and Web of Science clearly indicate some articles that have been retracted, but the vast majority go unrecorded even on these databases. Perhaps this is why even highly publicised retractions continue to be cited by articles that follow (Piller, 2021). Clearly, the community is still responsible for watching what happens to the literature, even once a paper is cited. Of course, the publishers could be using items such as DOIs to track retracted papers and query their citations. So why don't they?

Some literature databases will notify you if a paper that you have in your database is retracted – but don't count on this unless you use Zotero. Zotero takes DOIs from the retraction watch database, and uses them to notify any retractions of articles that have occurred. A large red bar (that's hard to ignore) is shown across the top of the citation window. This is a strong and very positive reason for using Zotero.

Publishers are bad at sending through the correct metadata with their content. For example, for the same 30 year period as Figure 30.1, Web of Science lists only 133 retractions. Really what this means is that if you aren't using Zotero, and you want to be sure that there hasn't been a retraction in any of your source material, you need to run a search on the Retraction Watch database – "better to use Zotero", says Ivan Oransky. Right now, the chance that any paper published in the last 30 years that you have cited will get retracted is still low (1 in 1750), but if it was published in 2020 this rises to 1 in 650.

30.3.2 Notification of retraction

The notification of retraction is supposed to explain exactly why a paper has been retracted. For example, if you have cited or used this work you should know whether it is because data has been fabricated, or more innocently there was a mistake with the equipment or another aspect of the investigation. However, it seems that some journals are issuing retraction notices that fall short of the guidelines required by COPE (Barbour et al., 2009), and that these delays are not in the interest of anyone involved (see Grey et al., 2021;

Teixeira da Silva, 2021a). Clearly, there is need for improvement here on the part of the journals.

But we must be cautious about playing a blame game when it comes to journal retractions (Smith, 2021). We already know that peer review has shortcomings (see Part IV), and even the best of peer reviewers and/or editors cannot be expected to spot potentially fatal errors, especially when these come about from deliberate deceit on the part of the authors. Retraction will remain a necessary part of the scientific publishing process, and as retractions become more commonplace among journals, we can hope that guidelines will be followed in a timely manor (Grey et al., 2021).

30.4   Retraction Watch

To learn more about retractions in science, I encourage you to read the blog at Retraction Watch (retractionwatch.com). This will give you an idea of the reasons why retractions are made, and give you some perspectives about the practices (and malpractices) that go on in the scientific environment.

30.5   Fabrication of data

The fabrication of data does happen. An anonymous survey on research integrity in the Netherlands suggested that prevalence of fabrication was 4.3% and falsification was 4.2%, while nearly half of those surveyed admitted to questionable research practices most prevalent in PhD candidates and junior researchers (Golpalakrishna et al., 2021).

A growing body of retractions and alleged evidence on the tampering of data in spreadsheets has led to the suspension of a top Canadian researcher, Jonathan Pruitt. The detection of fraudulent (usually duplicated) data in spreadsheets is not too difficult to spot (e.g. by application of Benford's law – the last digits of naturally occurring numbers should approach uniformity), and has become the subject of some contract data scientists who specialise in finding such instances of fraud. To some extent, the automated assessment of fraudulent practices has been or could be implemented for many infringements (Bordewijk et al., 2021).

The existence of paper mills should also be mentioned at this point. Papers, produced commercially and to order, are entirely fabricated by third parties to improve the CVs of real paying scientists (Teixeira da Silva, 2021a; Byrne, 2019). Hundreds of these papers have been discovered that appear to come from the same source (Bik, 2020), but the true size of such additions to the scientific literature is unknown.

The pressure to publish is widely acknowledged as driving questionable research practices, including fraud (Golpalakrishna et al., 2021). Some have suggested that the pressure to obtain a permanent academic position is enough to drive some scientists to commit fraud (Husemann et al., 2017; Kun, 2018; Fanelli et al., 2015). The idiom 'publish or perish', and the importance of publishing is made elsewhere. However, I hope that by shedding some light on unethical practices, this book equips you to avoid these together with those that may espouse them, and instead show you that there is a better path to success.

Pruitt's case (see below) highlights a good reason for increased transparency in the publication process. A blog post from someone caught up in the Pruitt retractions makes the point that journals that insisted on full data deposits for publication were well ahead of those that hadn't (Bolnick, 2021). Of growing concern in many areas of Biological Sciences is the potential to manipulate results that are essentially images, for example blots on a gel. However, it turns out that manipulated images are also not too hard to discern.

Images are increasingly being used in journals to demonstrate results, and the manipulation of images in published papers appears to be rife. In a study of more than 20,000 papers from 40 journals (1995 to 2014), Bik et al. (2016) found that nearly 2% had features suggesting deliberate manipulation. These could include simple duplication of an image from supposedly different experiments, duplication with manipulation (e.g. rotation, reversal, etc.) and duplication with alteration (including adding and subtracting parts of the copied image). The authors suggested that as they only considered these types of manipulations from certain image types, the actual level of image fraud in scientific papers is likely much higher (Bik et al., 2016). An R package (FraudDetTools) is now available for checking manipulation of images (Koppers et al., 2017), but there are other steps that reviewers and editors can take themselves (Byrne and Christopher, 2020).

30.5.1 Who is responsible?

In the case of fraud, retraction statements should indicate who the perpetrator is in order to exonerate the other researchers. Some research into the likely source of the fraud has been conducted. There are clearly serial fraudsters, and the presence of their names in the author list is a red flag for those investigating fraud. Data from papers that are known to be fraudulent suggest that the first author is the most likely to be responsible for the fraud committed, and middle authors the least (Hussinger and Pellens, 2019). This suggests that you should be very careful who you collaborate with. While you might not be responsible, the discovery of (particularly large scale) fraud might well harm your career.

A study looking for patterns about types of authors involved in retractions (all reasons), suggested that Early Career Researchers were particularly likely to be involved in retractions (Fanelli et al., 2015), although the exact reason why remains obscure.

It is worth noting that while the journals (and ultimately the journal editor) are responsible for retractions from journals, this is not the same as punishing individuals who have committed fraud. As we have already seen, there can be many reasons for a retraction, and it is not up to editors or journals to punish researchers as there will be innocent researchers who may also need to make retractions. Moreover, it should never be the role of the journal to have any punitive action over a researcher. There are other mechanisms for this with the employer and (where applicable) the academic society involved. Different institutions and governments will have different rules when it comes to fraud being committed by their employees. These processes may be legal and take some time to finish. As we will see with the case of Pruitt, once lawyers get involved, the process may become mired in a lot more bureaucracy.

Whilst you may consider that your employers are not a group that you are particularly concerned about, you should consider the possibility that any scientific fraud could penetrate deeper. For example, if you used fraudulently fabricated data in order to make a grant application look better, then this would be deemed very serious by the (probable) government granting body that you were applying to. Essentially, this becomes financial fraud as you are using false data in order to obtain money. While your employers may simply remove you from your position (and their employment), the government might prosecute and you could find yourself in prison. This does happen in some countries, and so (obviously) it is a really bad idea to commit fraud.

30.6   What to do if you suspect others

If you suspect that someone in a lab in your department, faculty or university is fabricating data, find out whether your university has a research integrity officer (RIO); most universities in the US have one. Document your evidence if you can and approach the RIO or person in the equivalent position. If you can't find such a person, then ask at your university library for the most relevant person. Libraries are usually neutral places where you can find out information without arousing suspicion. You do need to be careful that you do not place yourself in harm's way when reporting, so be prudent about sharing until you are assured protection from any potential retaliation. It isn't easy to be a whistleblower – but it is the right thing to do.

If the research is published, and you think it is fraudulent, approach the editor directly. If there is some conflict of interest (like the person is at your institution), then you can try to sort it out internally (as described above). Otherwise, you can approach the editor directly yourself, anonymously or by using a third party.

COPE has published some useful flowcharts to guide researchers who suspect fraud in manuscripts or published articles:

- 'Image manipulation in a published article' (COPE, 2018c)
- 'How to recognise potential authorship problems' (COPE, 2018a)
- 'Systematic manipulation of the publication process' (COPE, 2018b)
- 'How to recognise potential manipulation of the peer review process' (COPE, 2017)
- 'If you suspect fabricated data in a submitted manuscript' (Wager, 2006a)
- 'Ghost, guest, or gift authorship in a submitted manuscript' (Wager, 2006b)
- Undisclosed conflict of interest
    - in a submitted manuscript
    - in a published article
- 'Plagiarism in a submitted manuscript' (Wager, 2006c)

30.7 Confirmation bias and the paradox of high-flying academic careers

Jonathan Pruitt had it all going for him. His studies of spider sociality were producing novel and significant results that opened the door to publications in high impact journals. In turn, this opened the door to getting prizes and funding. The funding allowed him to conduct more studies and soon a prestigious chair in Canada with more funding to pursue his rocketing career. Things started to unravel for Pruitt when colleagues raised concern about the data in some of his publications. Things gathered pace very quickly, and doubt gathered around more and more of his publications. Although there is much written about the

Pruitt debacle on the internet, the blog by *American Naturalist* editor and former Pruitt fan and friend, Dan Bolnick, is particularly enlightening (Bolnick, 2021). Pruitt's case is becoming increasingly untenable as more editors backed by co-authors are retracting papers where he contributed data (see Marcus, 2020). For Pruitt, this has become a threat to his career and livelihood (Pennisi, 2020). Similarly, his university is facing the possibility that they hired a fraud. Consequently, this whole debacle has slipped into the legal world. Bolnick has clearly suffered personally from the affair, but has set out to provide as transparent an account as possible.

The harrowing part of Bolnick's account is when he, co-authors and other editors started to receive letters from Pruitt's lawyer (see Bolnick, 2021, for one example). At the point that the lawyer steps in, the functioning academic community that had raised itself to meet the demands of the concerns began to get muted. Bolnick then makes an important point that the legal threats from Pruitt's lawyer were stifling the freedom for academics (in this case the co-authors and editors) to publish, and therefore their academic freedom.

Another example of a rising star with high profile papers, allegedly making a habit of fabricating data, comes from the world of marine biology (Clark et al., 2020). The researchers in question, Danielle Dixson under the supervision of Philip Munday, made counter-claims that the detractors were unimaginative or that they are attempting to make a career from criticism. Meanwhile, students from their own labs continue to raise concern about the culture of fraud (see Enserink, 2021). In this case, the tide of evidence against the marine biologists appears to have turned, with forensic data specialists finding multiple examples of suspect data.

Neither case is fully resolved as the cases against these scientists still rest with their institutions. The lives of co-authors, former students and colleagues are put on hold, until some unforeseen point in the future.

It is clear from these reports that there are systemic problems when high profile scientists are accused of fraud. Journals say that it's the responsibility of the institutions, and the institutions have no impetus to find fraud as that might lose a very productive (think research income) and high profile scientist. What university would want to have its name dragged through the mud, and on top of this lose a large amount of grant income? Top researchers become untouchables in many institutions because they are essentially cash cows that no-one wants to disturb. Allegations against such individuals also include bullying and sexual misconduct. For those interested in reading more high profile misdemeaners in science Stuart Ritchie (2020) has put together a popular book on the subject.

Another important issue that arises from (alleged) scientific fraud is that it creates a culture of research that pushes towards an extremely unlikely hypothesis, in the misbelief that the hypothesis is likely given the nature of the publications (also see Fanelli et al., 2017). Indeed, this natural selection of 'bad science' has permeated the hiring system so that researchers like this are more likely to be hired (Smaldino and McElreath, 2016). Forsmeier et al. (2017) have an excellent review that outlines the problems with a culture that pushes towards increasingly unlikely hypotheses (see also Measey, 2021, on Type I errors).

At the heart of all of this is the cult of the Impact Factor and the research mentality that it generates.

31

Are you bullying or being bullied?

I am going to write here about academic bullying because it is currently prevalent in academia, and because most of the bullies are unaware of what they are doing. In a 2019 survey of graduate students (see Woolston, 2019; Figure 31.1), 22% felt that they had experienced bullying during their PhD program. The only way of improving the situation around academic bullying is for everyone to become more aware. It may not be happening to you, but it may be happening to people around you either in your lab or in another lab in the same department or faculty. If you think that this is very rare behaviour in academia, think again (Devlin and Marsh, 2018).

31.1   How to spot a bully

A bully is anyone who abuses or misuses their position of power in order to humiliate, denigrate or injure another. This does not need to be or someone in your lab. It can be anyone in your working environment (watch the video here[1] or here[2]) including people in your institutes' administration. These people are usually in positions of power with influence over you and your future. As in my example (below) you may be worried that the power they have could be used by them to negatively impact your future. If you are worried about this, then their behaviour most likely conforms to bullying. Bullying often involves harassment that is designed to undermine your dignity, often through sexism, racism, or another prejudice (Krishna and Soumyaja, 2020). Even if you think that your bully didn't mean to cause offence, the fact that they did upset you and that this behaviour was unwanted is enough to fulfil the criteria for bullying. Thus, it is not what they intended, but what you felt that is important in bullying. A direct consequence of this is that bullies often don't recognise this as a description of their behaviour. It is worth bearing in mind that bullies are often damaged individuals who are repeating

---

[1] https://youtu.be/bZmmp7i9Tsc
[2] https://youtu.be/lKUONMm-pWo

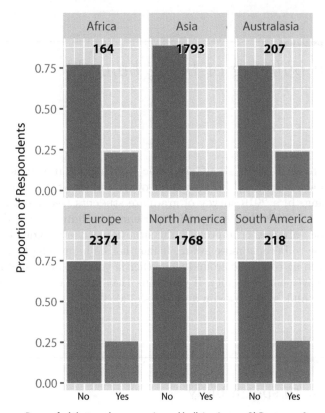

Do you feel that you have experienced bullying in your PhD program?

FIGURE 31.1: Do you feel that you have experienced bullying in your PhD program? Responses to a survey of graduate students demonstrate the changes in bullying propensity in different research cultures. Survey data taken from 2019 *Nature* survey (see Woolston, 2019).

behaviour that they have themselves experienced from others. This doesn't excuse their behaviour, but they may think that such behaviour is normal.

What you should ask yourself is if someone were to observe this behaviour from the outside, would they recognise the interaction as normal or see that something was not correct? Of course, if you observe this going on with someone else in your group, or outside your group. Take the initiative to approach the person after and determine whether they feel like a victim: remember that not all interactions are as they appear from the outside. This is where a good set of institutional rules about bullying is important.

31.2   What to do about bullying

First, you need to find the rules that your institution has regarding bullying. If your institution has no rules, then they will need them and so helping them achieve this would be a good place to start (Mahmoudi and Keashly, 2021). No one wants to be the first case study, but there may need to be a first in order to set up a protocol.

Avoid the bully when asking for your institutional rules, but you should be able to find them via your departmental secretary, administrative support staff in the department or faculty. Read the documentation carefully and learn about how and by whom such reports are dealt with. Become aware of resources that are available – paritymovement.org is a great place to start. Read more about other people's experiences and be aware that you are not alone (Mahmoudi, 2020; Malaga-Trillo and Gerlach, 2004).

Next, document your case. Make some notes about the incident(s), when they happened, what was said, how you were made to feel, and what power you feel the person has over you.

Share your burden with a trusted friend or colleague. It is worth sharing the incident with others to see what they think about your predicament. In the survey mentioned above, more than half of the respondents who said that they experienced bullying felt that they could not discuss their experience for fear of reprisals. However, you do not have to discuss it inside the workplace, and often it's better to talk to people outside as the context is not so important in bullying. In your description, attempt to strip down the interaction into the component parts.

Follow your university's rules about who to go to with your complaint. Don't leave it to the next person in your lab to experience, they may not be as strong or as resourceful as you. It may not be your career that is destroyed, and the next student might not be so lucky.

31.3   What to do if the procedure against bullying at your institution doesn't work

My worst experience of bullying happened when I was a PhD student. It happened to me, and I witnessed it happening to other members of my lab. It wasn't hard to spot. Students would come out of my advisor's office in tears, and recount horrific stories of how he had debased and humiliated them. At the time, our department had no specific code on bullying, but there was a complaints procedure which started with the head of department. Unfortunately, as my advisor was also the head of the department, I could not follow the procedure as it was supposed to be done. Instead, I went to the academic who was responsible for postgraduates. The first two times, that staff member simply went to the head of department (yes, my advisor) and I was called in both times and bullied some more: how dare I complain about him?

The last time I tried to complain, once I had finished my PhD and felt much safer from the bully, I went to the dean of the faculty. He was the line manager of my advisor (still head of department) and was a lot more sympathetic. After listening to my story, and how my other lab mates were still suffering, he called them in one by one. And one by one they each denied all of the bullying that had happened. They were afraid. Unlike me, who had finished, they were still relying on their advisor to get their postgraduate degrees. The result was that without any corroborating evidence, there was no case for the dean to take forward.

What should you do if the procedure at your institution doesn't work? You become a survivor. You also become more vigilant against bullying in the future. Whatever happens, don't be tempted to become the bully yourself. Support other survivors and make progress to improve the system for future postgraduate students. Bullying is in human nature, and it won't stop. But we can make people more aware of it, and we can have procedures that work both for the bullied and the bullies.

32

Keeping track of your mental health

Stress is a natural part of life, and many people are at their most productive when they are under some degree of pressure, such as a deadline. Although deadlines don't work for everyone. Problems arise when we become overwhelmed by stress and are unable to fully respond. When this occurs, productivity can drop off and survival responses can be triggered as if responding to an actual physical attack. These responses include fight, flight or freeze responses. Anxiety and panic can be triggered. In this state additional demands on your time may also push your life off balance, so that you start to neglect your personal wellbeing which can negatively impact on relationships, exercise regime, or even nutrition and personal hygiene. Some people can find that the additional stress can cause physical symptoms that may even need medical treatment. Your sense of competence and mastery can be negatively impacted such that you may even suffer from feelings of inadequacy or imposter syndrome. Impostor syndrome is an experience you have when you believe that you are not as competent as you think others perceive you to be. It is not uncommon in many professions, and especially prevalent in academia (Clance and Imes, 1978). This is now widely recognised and there are lots of useful shared experiences out there to read (e.g. Dickerson, 2019; Woolston, 2016).

The General Health Questionnaire is an instrument used to measure psychological distress. For example, you could use the GHQ-12 (given in Table 4.1[1] of Measey, 2021). It is quick, reliable and simple to score, so you can use it at any time during your career as an indicator of whether you need to reach out to personal, occupational or professional support networks. My suggestion is that you complete a General Health Questionnaire now and record your answers as a baseline. Keep the scores somewhere safe. If you feel that you are getting overly stressed, take the test again and compare them with your baseline scores. Although there are no hard rules, if three or more of your scores have moved by two or more points it could be worth discussing with your support network to help you decide whether or not to seek professional help.

Even if you don't feel you need the support of your institution now, it is worth finding out how they can support your mental health in the future if needed. Although there has been some stigma attached to difficulties with mental

---

[1] http://www.howtowriteaphd.org/healthy.html#tab:GHQ

DOI: 10.1201/9781003220886-32

health in the past, most institutions accept that pressures are mounting on their staff and that they may require support. Most institutions will make experienced councillors available to support you if needed. Importantly, you should realise that none of these symptoms are unusual and that there is a high probability that many of your colleagues may also be struggling. Knowing that your problems are shared and reaching out to support networks early is an excellent way to prevent them from escalating beyond your control. Your best means of coping will be to try and develop a support network and to understand where and with whom you can discuss any difficulties as they arise. Knowing who this is and how and when to approach them will put you in a stronger position if you need them in future.

32.1   Being physically active improves mental wellbeing

The positive relationship between the amount of physical activity and higher mental wellbeing is well established (e.g. Grasdalsmoen et al. 2020; Gerber et al. 2014), but the kind of exercise required to achieve this improved result is varied. There are plenty of studies out there that suggest there are multiple benefits from physical activity (Williams, 2021). This does not have to be the most hectic exercise possible. You'll get huge benefits from simply taking a walk.

Exercise does not exclude you from participating in other less physical activities, including mindfulness or meditation. Try different types of activities and then do what's right for you.

Use the time that you spend exercising as thinking time: turn ideas over in your head, think through the logic in arguments, and potential flaws in experimental design. If you can, spend this moving time with others in your group discussing projects and talking about ideas. There are reasons why we do some of our best thinking when physically active, and you should seek to exploit these when you can. For example, if you have a meeting scheduled then why not do it as a walk – even if it's on the university campus this walk will get you and your colleague in a much better space to plan ideas.

This isn't to say that you won't need time at the computer writing it all down, or talking around a table with colleagues. Be inventive in how you spend your time, and don't resign yourself to spending all day sitting behind a desk. Don't take my word for it, see this great new book by Caroline Williams (2021).

33

Habilitation, DSc and Tenure

These are qualifications post-PhD that exist in some countries and might be prerequisites to getting some positions within academia. I do not go into these in detail here because they are country specific, and you are likely to learn much more about them at your own institution. The brief inclusion here serves as a guide to their existence, and for you to be aware that different rules apply in different countries, and that if you are mobile in your career there may be additional steps that are required of you before you can apply for a job or certain promotions.

33.1   Habilitation

Habilitation from the Latin *habilitare*, 'to make fit', started in Germany first as part of the PhD process, and later as a separate post-doctoral qualification in the 1800s. This process has been adopted by a number of (mostly European) countries as a requisite step in teaching or directing research. In countries where this qualification exists, it is usually a prerequisite before being able to apply as a candidate for a professorship. In some countries, most notably Germany, the habilitation comes after having already held a job as a researcher and lecturer, and comes with a serious expectation that this will lead to a promotion to become a professor. In this way, it could be seen as a similar process to going for tenure in the US.

In France, the related qualification is the Habilitation à Diriger des Recherches (Accreditation to Direct Research or HDR). Like the German system, the HDR is applied for by someone who already holds a position as a lecturer (Maître de Conférences) for several years, when they hold sufficient research to put together a portfolio. You need to be accredited with HDR before you can advise PhD students. Ironically, this portfolio should include the supervision of at least one PhD student. Thus, you'll need to arrange to be a co-advisor when you are actually the main advisor, before moving forward with your HDR portfolio. Given that your first PhD student may take some years to

DOI: 10.1201/9781003220886-33

finish, it would be worth finding a sympathetic person with an HDR sooner rather than later, once you are in your Maître de Conférences post.

In the Biological Sciences, most requirements for habilitation are cumulative, meaning that you can assemble a set of published research papers that you have written or led. The number and quality of such publications will depend on where you are submitting this thesis, meaning that in some places it may take as long as 10 years. Importantly, the habilitation is not advised.

33.2   Doctor of Science (DSc)

In the absence of any requirement for habilitation, there is the possibility (at many universities) of compiling published papers, that you have written or directed, into a thesis that can be examined for a Doctor of Science (DSc). Like the PhD, the DSc allows you to call yourself Doctor (although you likely already can) and put the letters DSc after your name. The DSc is touted as an advanced doctoral degree. You will need to register as you would for a PhD, but in most cases your thesis will not be advised.

One interesting point to note is that registration for a DSc need not have possession of a PhD as a prerequisite. If you are in a position where you have never done a PhD, but have worked within or alongside academia, including publishing papers, for a considerable period, you might be in a position to register for a DSc.

33.3   Tenure

Obtaining tenure (in the USA and Canada and some other countries) gives you a special kind of academic freedom such that it is very hard for you to be removed from your post. In some states this means that you are not required to retire: a job for life – although there are increasingly attractive offers for professors to retire (Campbell, 2016; Nakada and Xu, 2018). Tenure exists around the need for independent academic freedom: that as an academic scholar you are free to hold your own, scholarly views, and as such cannot be censured by the state. Getting tenure, therefore, at the university where you are employed is an important step, vital if you want to move from contract to permanent employment. In practice, if you don't get tenure it will most likely mean that you won't get to continue at that university: tenure or bust.

In order to obtain tenure in most US universities you will need to provide:

- A portfolio of peer-reviewed published research
- The proven ability to attract grant funding
  - A significant amount of which goes to the university
- Teaching excellence
  - As assessed by undergraduate and postgraduate students
- Academic visibility
  - The recognition of your research by peers through inclusion in conferences, invitations to give seminars, etc.
- Administrative and/or community service
  - This includes roles such as being an editor for a journal
  - Peer review for journals and grant awarding bodies
  - Serving on your university's committees and panels

The relative importance to each of the above aspects will depend on the type of college where you are trying to get tenure. Unsurprisingly, a teaching college will require you to have excellence in teaching, while a research university will place more emphasis on your research portfolio and your standing as an academic in the international community. If you aren't from North America, it is important that you know what the priorities of your institution are before you apply for a position there, or even before you try to do a postgraduate degree.

Once you are in an untenured post at a US university, you will have a limited amount of time to achieve the above portfolio in order to apply for tenure. Getting tenure often comes together with promotion (to professor) and a reduction in (undergraduate) teaching load. The time limited nature of getting tenure is such that even after you have received your PhD, this is a much higher hurdle to attain.

Last note

I really hope that this book has been helpful and that it has achieved what I set out to do: provide you with the guide on how to publish in the Biological Sciences. If you feel that this book has important items missing, is out-of-date or simply wrong, then please contribute. Any good guide relies upon the people who use it to keep it viable. My special plea to those of you who are Early Career Researchers is to become part of the solution for shifting from the closed to open models of scientific publishing. In doing so, you will make science more transparent, open and equitable. While there is much that is currently wrong in the system, the vast majority of the actors in it are working for the good of science. While I conceded that publishing science is a wicked problem which is not easily solved, there are some simple steps that we can all make towards a resolution that benefits science.

When seeking a solution to publishing science, and publishing in other academic disciplines, we cannot compromise on the cornerstones of the scientific method: **rigour, independence, transparency and reproducibility**. This book should have highlighted aspects of scientific publishing that currently violate these cornerstones and so need to be changed. When you can, select those journals and publishers that maintain the highest standards. Join your discipline's academic society and stand for election to a position. Issue your clarion call for change. Join the gatekeepers of the society's journals, and use your soft power to help bring about change.

1. Make more use of archiving services: preprints, data and proposals
2. Make use of independent peer review services: peer community in, and peer commons
3. Persuade your society to move to a Diamond Open Access overlay journal model
4. Become part of the solution, start an Open Science Community in your institution

Bibliography

Abdill, R. J. and Blekhman, R. (2019). Tracking the popularity and outcomes of all bioRxiv preprints. *eLife*, 8:e45133.

Adam, D. (2002). The counting house. *Nature*, 415(6873):726–729.

Adams, J. (2012). The rise of research networks. *Nature*, 490(7420):335–336.

Aksnes, D. W. (2003). A macro study of self-citation. *Scientometrics*, 56(2):235–246.

Armeni, K. Brinkman, L., Carlsson, R., Eerland, A., Fijten, R., Fondberg, R., Heininga V.E., et al. (2021) "Towards Wide-Scale Adoption of Open Science Practices: The Role of Open Science Communities." *Science and Public Policy* 48, scab039-. https://doi.org/10.1093/scipol/scab039.

Anderson, J., Nicholas, S., and Smith, P. (2021). Campaign to investigate the academic ebook market. https://academicebookinvestigation.org/.

Anderson, K. (2021). Altmetric Devalues Twitter, Tells Nobody. https://thegeyser.substack.com/p/altmetric-quietly-devalues-twitter.

Anderson, M. S., Martinson, B. C., and De Vries, R. (2007). Normative dissonance in science: Results from a national survey of US scientists. *Journal of Empirical Research on Human Research Ethics*, 2(4):3–14.

Anon (2018). Retraction. *Behavioral Ecology*, 29(2):508–508.

Baglini, R. and Parsons, C. (2020). If you can't be kind in peer review, be neutral. Nature Careers Community https://doi.org/10.1038/d41586-020-03394-y.

Baker, M. (2016). 1,500 scientists lift the lid on reproducibility : Nature News & Comment. *Nature*, 533:452–454.

Baković, E. (2017). Language Log » More Zombie Lingua shenanigans. https://languagelog.ldc.upenn.edu/nll/?p=34106.

Bar-Ilan, J. and Halevi, G. (2017). Post retraction citations in context: a case study. *Scientometrics*, 113(1):547–565.

Barbour, V., Kleinert, S., Wager, E., and Yentis, S. (2009). Guidelines for retracting articles. Technical report, Committee on Publication Ethics.

Barnett, A., Mewburn, I., and Schroter, S. (2019). Working 9 to 5, not the way to make an academic living: observational analysis of manuscript and peer review submissions over time. *BMJ*, 367:l6460.

Baskin, P. K. and Gross, R. A. (2011). Honorary and ghost authorship. *BMJ*, 343:d6223.

Baxter-Gilbert, J., Riley, J. L., Wagener, C., Mohanty, N. P., and Measey, J. (2020). Shrinking before our isles: the rapid expression of insular dwarfism in two invasive populations of guttural toad (*Sclerophrys gutturalis*). *Biology Letters*, 16(11):20200651.

Berenbaum, M. R. (2021). Editorial Expression of Concern: New class of transcription factors controls flagellar assembly by recruiting RNA polymerase II in Chlamydomonas. *Proceedings of the National Academy of Sciences*, 118(24).

Bergstrom, C. T. and Bergstrom, T. C. (2006). The economics of ecology journals. *Frontiers in Ecology and the Environment*, 4(9):488–495.

Bett, H. K. (2020). Predatory publishing through McCornarck's information manipulation theory. *Global Knowledge, Memory and Communication*, 69(4/5):331–339.

Bik, E. M. (2020). The Tadpole Paper Mill. https://scienceintegritydigest.com/2020/02/21/the-tadpole-paper-mill/.

Bik, E. M., Casadevall, A., and Fang, F. C. (2016). The Prevalence of Inappropriate Image Duplication in Biomedical Research Publications. *mBio*, 7(3):e00809–16.

Björk, B.-C. and Solomon, D. (2015). Article processing charges in OA journals: relationship between price and quality. *Scientometrics*, 103(2):373–385.

Bolnick, D. (2021). 17 months. https://ecoevoevoeco.blogspot.com/2021/05/17-months.html.

Bonnet, X., Shine, R., and Lourdais, O. (2002). Taxonomic chauvinism. *Trends in Ecology & Evolution*, 17(1):1–3.

Bordewijk, E. M., Li, W., Eekelen, R. v., Wang, R., Showell, M., Mol, B. W., and Wely, M. v. (2021). Methods to assess research misconduct in health-related research: A scoping review. *Journal of Clinical Epidemiology*, 136:189–202. https://doi.org/10.1016/j.jclinepi.2021.05.012.

Bornmann, L. and Marx, W. (2012). The Anna Karenina principle: A way of thinking about success in science. *Journal of the American Society for Information Science and Technology*, 63(10):2037–2051. _eprint: https://onlinelibrary.wiley.com/doi/pdf/10.1002/asi.22661.

Bornmann, L., Mutz, R., and Haunschild, R. (2020). Growth rates of modern science: A latent piecewise growth curve approach to model publication numbers from established and new literature databases. *arXiv preprint arXiv:2012.07675*.

Bornmann, L., Wolf, M., and Daniel, H.-D. (2012). Closed versus open reviewing of journal manuscripts: how far do comments differ in language use? *Scientometrics*, 91(3):843–856.

Brainard, J. and You, J. (2018). What a massive database of retracted papers reveals about science publishing's 'death penalty'. *Science*. https://www.sciencemag.org/news/2018/10/what-massive-database-retracted-papers-reveals-about-science-publishing-s-death-penalty.

Braun, T. and Dióspatonyi, I. (2005). Counting the gatekeepers of international science journals a worthwhile science indicator. *Current Science*, 89(9):1548–1551.

Bravo, G., Farjam, M., Moreno, F. G., Birukou, A., and Squazzoni, F. (2018). Hidden connections: Network effects on editorial decisions in four computer science journals. *Journal of Informetrics*, 12(1):101–112.

Brembs, B., Button, K., and Munafò, M. R. (2013). Deep impact: unintended consequences of journal rank. *Frontiers in Human Neuroscience*, 7:291.

Brembs, B., Huneman, P., Schönbrodt, F., Nilsonne, G., Susi, T., Siems, R., Perakakis, P., Trachana, V., Ma, L., and Rodriguez-Cuadrado, S. (2021). Replacing Academic Journals. *Zenodo*, September 24, 2021. https://doi.org/10.5281/zenodo.5526635.

Brock, W. H. (1980). The development of commercial science journals in Victorian Britain. *Development of science publishing in Europe*, pages 95–122.

Brown, J. (2010). An introduction to overlay journals. Report, Repositories Support Project, UK. http://www.rsp.ac.uk/pubs/.

Budden, A. E., Tregenza, T., Aarssen, L. W., Koricheva, J., Leimu, R., and Lortie, C. J. (2008). Double-blind review favours increased representation of female authors. *Trends in Ecology & Evolution*, 23(1):4–6.

Budzinski, O., Grebel, T., Wolling, J., and Zhang, X. (2020). Drivers of article processing charges in open access. *Scientometrics*, 124(3):2185–2206.

Buranyi, S. (2017). Is the staggeringly profitable business of scientific publishing bad for science? *The Guardian*. https://www.theguardian.com/science/2017/jun/27/profitable-business-scientific-publishing-bad-for-science.

Byrne, J. (2019). We Need to Talk about Systematic Fraud. Nature 566, no. 7742: 9-9. https://doi.org/10.1038/d41586-019-00439-9.

Byrne, J. A. and Christopher, J. (2020). Digital magic, or the dark arts of the 21st century—how can journals and peer reviewers detect manuscripts and publications from paper mills? *FEBS Letters*, 594(4):583–589. _eprint: https://febs.onlinelibrary.wiley.com/doi/pdf/10.1002/1873-3468.13747.

Campbell, A. F. (2016). The Workforce that Won't Retire. https://www.theatlantic.com/business/archive/2016/06/colleges-offer-retirement-buyouts-to-professors/487400/.

Casadevall, A. and Fang, F. C. (2012). Reforming Science: Methodological and Cultural Reforms. *Infection and Immunity*, 80(3):891–896.

Casnici, N., Grimaldo, F., Gilbert, N., Dondio, P., and Squazzoni, F. (2017). Assessing peer review by gauging the fate of rejected manuscripts: the case of the Journal of Artificial Societies and Social Simulation. *Scientometrics*, 113(1):533–546.

Cassey, P. and Blackburn, T. M. (2003). Publication rejection among ecologists. *Trends in Ecology & Evolution*, 18(8):375–376.

Cassey, P. and Blackburn, T. M. (2004). Publication and Rejection among Successful Ecologists. *BioScience*, 54(3):234–239.

Ceci, S. J. and Peters, D. P. (1982). Peer Review: A Study of Reliability. *Change*, 14(6):44–48.

Chapman, C. A., Bicca-Marques, J.C., Calvignac-Spencer, S., Fan, P., Fashing, P.J., Gogarten, J., Guo, S., et al. (2019). Games Academics Play and Their Consequences: How Authorship, h-Index and Journal Impact Factors Are Shaping the Future of Academia. *Proceedings of the Royal Society B: Biological Sciences 286*, 1916: 20192047. https://doi.org/10.1098/rspb.2019.2047.

Chawla, D. S. (2021). Scientists at odds on Utrecht University reforms to hiring and promotion criteria. https://www.natureindex.com/news-blog/scientists-argue-over-use-of-impact-factors-for-evaluating-research.

Cho, A. H., Johnson, S. A., Schuman, C. E., Adler, J. M., Gonzalez, O., Graves, S. J., Huebner, J. R., Marchant, D. B., Rifai, S. W., Skinner, I., and Bruna, E. M. (2014). Women are underrepresented on the editorial boards of journals in environmental biology and natural resource management. *PeerJ*, 2:e542.

Chorus, C. and Waltman, L. (2016). A Large-Scale Analysis of Impact Factor Biased Journal Self-Citations. *PLOS ONE*, 11(8):e0161021.

Christl, W. (2021). "Digitale Überwachung und Kontrolle am Arbeitsplatz. Von der Ausweitung betrieblicher Datenerfassung zum algorithmischen Management?" Cracked Labs, September 15, 2021. https://crackedlabs.org/daten-arbeitsplatz.

Christie, A. P., White, T. B., Martin, P., Petrovan, S. O., Bladon, A. J., Bowkett, A. E., Littlewood, N. A., Mupepele, A.-C., Rocha, R., Sainsbury, K. A., Smith, R. K., Taylor, N. G., and Sutherland, W. J. (2021). Reducing publication delay to improve the efficiency and impact of conservation science. *bioRxiv*, page 2021.03.30.437223. https://www.biorxiv.org/content/10.1101/2021.03.30.437223v2.

Clance, P. R. and Imes, S. A. (1978). The imposter phenomenon in high achieving women: Dynamics and therapeutic intervention. *Psychotherapy: Theory, Research & Practice*, 15(3):241–247.

Clark, T. D., Raby, G. D., Roche, D. G., Binning, S. A., Speers-Roesch, B., Jutfelt, F., and Sundin, J. (2020). Ocean acidification does not impair the behaviour of coral reef fishes. *Nature*, 577(7790):370–375.

COPE (2017). How to spot potential manipulation of the peer review process. Technical report, Committee on Publication Ethics. https://publicationethics.org/node/34311.

COPE (2018a). How to recognise potential authorship problems. Technical report, Committee on Publication Ethics. https://publicationethics.org/node/39531.

COPE (2018b). Systematic manipulation of the publication process. Technical report, Committee on Publication Ethics and Springer Nature. https://publicationethics.org/node/39471.

COPE (2018c). What to do if you suspect image manipulation in a published article. Technical report, Committee on Publication Ethics and Springer Nature. https://publicationethics.org/node/39536.

Crane, D. (1967). The Gatekeepers of Science: Some Factors Affecting the Selection of Articles for Scientific Journals. *The American Sociologist*, 2(4):195–201.

Crew, B. (2019). Here's how to deal with failure, say senior scientists. https://www.natureindex.com/news-blog/how-to-deal-with-failure-rejection-academic-research-say-senior-scientists.

Crijns, T. J., Ottenhoff, J. S. E., and Ring, D. (2021). The effect of peer review on the improvement of rejected manuscripts. *Accountability in Research*, 28(8):517–527. https://doi.org/10.1080/08989621.2020.1869547.

Cronin, B. (2001). Hyperauthorship: A postmodern perversion or evidence of a structural shift in scholarly communication practices? *Journal of the American Society for Information Science and Technology*, 52(7):558–569.

Davarpanah, M. R. and Amel, F. (2009). Author self-citation pattern in science. *Library Review*, 58(4):301–309.

Davies, P. (2019). Is PLOS Running Out Of Time? Financial Statements Suggest Urgency To Innovate. https://scholarlykitchen.sspnet.org/2019/11/22/is-plos-running-out-of-time/.

Davies, S. W., Putnam, H. M., Ainsworth, T., Baum, J. K., Bove, C. B., Crosby, S. C., Côté, I. M., Duplouy, A., Fulweiler, R. W., Griffin, A. J., Hanley, T. C., Hill, T., Humanes, A., Mangubhai, S., Metaxas, A., Parker, L. M., Rivera, H. E., Silbiger, N. J., Smith, N. S., Spalding, A. K., Traylor-Knowles, N., Weigel, B. L., Wright, R. M., and Bates, A. E. (2021). Promoting inclusive metrics of success and impact to dismantle a discriminatory reward system in science. *PLOS Biology*, 19(6):e3001282.

Day, N. E. (2011). The Silent Majority: Manuscript Rejection and Its Impact on Scholars. *Academy of Management Learning & Education*, 10(4):704–718.

Demeter, M. (2018). Changing Center and Stagnant Periphery in Communication and Media Studies: National Diversity of Major International Journals in the Field of Communication from 2013 to 2017. *International Journal of Communication*, 12(1):29.

Deutz, D. B., Drachen, T. M., Drongstrup, D., Opstrup, N., and Wien, C. (2021). Quantitative quality: a study on how performance-based measures may change the publication patterns of Danish researchers. *Scientometrics*, 126(4):3303–3320.

Devlin, H. and Marsh, S. (2018). Hundreds of academics at top UK universities accused of bullying. *the Guardian*. http://www.theguardian.com/education/2018/sep/28/academics-uk-universities-accused-bullying-students-colleagues.

Dickerson, D. (2019). How I overcame impostor syndrome after leaving academia. *Nature*, 574(7779):588–588.

Dondio, P., Casnici, N., Grimaldo, F., Gilbert, N., and Squazzoni, F. (2019). The "invisible hand" of peer review: The implications of author-referee networks on peer review in a scholarly journal. *Journal of Informetrics*, 13(2):708–716.

Drvenica, I., Bravo, G., Vejmelka, L., Dekanski, A., and Nedić, O. (2019). Peer Review of Reviewers: The Author's Perspective. *Publications*, 7(1):1. https://www.mdpi.com/2304-6775/7/1/1.

Ducarme, F., Luque, G., and Courchamp, F. (2013). What are "charismatic species" for conservation biologists? *BioSciences Master Reviews*, 1:1–8.

Egghe, L. (2006). Theory and practise of the g-index. *Scientometrics*, 69(1):131–152.

Eisen, M. B., Akhmanova, A., Behrens, T. E., Harper, D. M., Weigel, D., and Zaidi, M. (2020). Implementing a "publish, then review" model of publishing. *eLife*, 9:e64910.

Ellender, B. and Weyl, O. (2014). A review of current knowledge, risk and ecological impacts associated with non-native freshwater fish introductions in South Africa. *Aquatic Invasions*, 9(2):117–132.

Else, H. (2021). Open-access publisher PLOS pushes to extend clout beyond biomedicine. *Nature*, 593(7860):489–490.

Enserink, M. (2021). Does ocean acidification alter fish behavior? Fraud allegations create a sea of doubt. *Science*, 372(6542):560–565.

Eve, M. P., Neylon, C., O'Donnell, D. P., Moore, S., Gadie, R., Odeniyi, V., and Parvin, S. (2021). Reading Peer Review: PLOS ONE and Institutional Change in Academia. *Elements in Publishing and Book Culture*. Cambridge University Press.

Eysenbach, G. (2019). Celebrating 20 Years of Open Access and Innovation at JMIR Publications. *Journal of Medical Internet Research*, 21(12):e17578.

Fanelli, D. (2010). "Positive" results increase down the hierarchy of the sciences. *PLOS ONE*, 5(4):e10068.

Fanelli, D. (2012). Negative results are disappearing from most disciplines and countries. *Scientometrics*, 90(3):891–904.

Fanelli, D., Costas, R., and Ioannidis, J. P. A. (2017). Meta-assessment of bias in science. *Proceedings of the National Academy of Sciences*, 114(14):3714–3719.

Fanelli, D., Costas, R., and Larivière, V. (2015). Misconduct Policies, Academic Culture and Career Stage, Not Gender or Pressures to Publish, Affect Scientific Integrity. *PLOS ONE*, 10(6):e0127556.

Fanelli, D. and Larivière, V. (2016). Researchers' Individual Publication Rate Has Not Increased in a Century. *PLOS ONE*, 11(3):e0149504.

Fang, F. C., Bowen, A., and Casadevall, A. (2016). NIH peer review percentile scores are poorly predictive of grant productivity. *eLife*, 5:e13323.

Fang, F. C. and Casadevall, A. (2011). Retracted Science and the Retraction Index. *Infection and Immunity*, 79(10):3855–3859.

Fang, F. C. and Casadevall, A. (2012). Reforming Science: Structural Reforms. *Infection and Immunity*, 80(3):897–901.

Fang, F. C., Steen, R. G., and Casadevall, A. (2012). Misconduct accounts for the majority of retracted scientific publications. *Proceedings of the National Academy of Sciences*, 109(42):17028–17033.

Farji-Brener, A. G. and Kitzberger, T. (2014). Rejecting Editorial Rejections Revisited: Are Editors of Ecological Journals Good Oracles? *The Bulletin of the Ecological Society of America*, 95(3):238–242.

Field, A. (2013). *Discovering Statistics Using IBM SPSS Statistics*. SAGE. London, UK.

Flatt, J. W., Blasimme, A., and Vayena, E. (2017). Improving the Measurement of Scientific Success by Reporting a Self-Citation Index. *Publications*, 5(3):20.

Forstmeier, W., Wagenmakers, E.-J., and Parker, T. H. (2017). Detecting and avoiding likely false-positive findings–a practical guide. *Biological Reviews*, 92(4):1941–1968.

Fortunato, S. Bergstrom, C.T., Börner, K., Evans, J.A., Helbing, D., Milojević, S., Petersen, A.M., et al. (2018). Science of Science. Science 359, 6379: eaao0185. https://doi.org/10.1126/science.aao0185.

Fowler, J. H. and Aksnes, D. W. (2007). Does self-citation pay? *Scientometrics*, 72(3):427–437.

Fox, C. W., Duffy, M. A., Fairbairn, D. J., and Meyer, J. A. (2019). Gender diversity of editorial boards and gender differences in the peer review process at six journals of ecology and evolution. *Ecology and Evolution*, 9(24):13636–13649.

Fox, C. W. and Paine, C. E. T. (2019). Gender differences in peer review outcomes and manuscript impact at six journals of ecology and evolution. *Ecology and Evolution*, 9(6):3599–3619.

Franco, A., Malhotra, N., and Simonovits, G. (2014). Publication bias in the social sciences: Unlocking the file drawer. *Science*, 345(6203):1502–1505.

Fuchs, C. and Sandoval, M. (2013). The Diamond Model of Open Access Publishing: Why Policy Makers, Scholars, Universities, Libraries, Labour Unions and the Publishing World Need to Take Non-Commercial, Non-Profit Open Access Serious. TripleC: Communication, Capitalism & Critique. 11, (2): 428–43. https://doi.org/10.31269/triplec.v11i2.502.

Galipeau, J., Barbour, V., Baskin, P., Bell-Syer, S., Cobey, K., Cumpston, M., Deeks, J., Garner, P., MacLehose, H., Shamseer, L., Straus, S., Tugwell, P., Wager, E., Winker, M., and Moher, D. (2016). A scoping review of competencies for scientific editors of biomedical journals. *BMC Medicine*, 14(1):16.

Garfield, E. (1999). Journal impact factor: a brief review. *CMAJ*, 161(8):979–980.

Garfunkel, J. M., Ulshen, M. H., Hamrick, H. J., and Lawson, E. E. (1994). Effect of Institutional Prestige on Reviewers' Recommendations and Editorial Decisions. *JAMA*, 272(2):137–138.

Glonti, K., Cauchi, D., Cobo, E., Boutron, I., Moher, D., and Hren, D. (2019). A scoping review on the roles and tasks of peer reviewers in the manuscript review process in biomedical journals. *BMC Medicine*, 17(1):118.

Gopalakrishna, G. ter Riet, G., Cruyff, M.J.L.F., Vink, G., Stoop, I., Wicherts, J., and Bouter, L. (2021). Prevalence of Questionable Research Practices, Research Misconduct and Their Potential Explanatory Factors: A Survey among Academic Researchers in The Netherlands. MetaArXiv, https://doi.org/10.31222/osf.io/vk9yt.

Goyanes, M. and Demeter, M. (2020). How the Geographic Diversity of Editorial Boards Affects What Is Published in JCR-Ranked Communication Journals. *Journalism & Mass Communication Quarterly*, 97(4):1123–1148.

Goyes Vallejos, J. (2021). What's in a name? *Science*, 372(6543):754–754.

Gray, R. J. (2020). Sorry, we're open: Golden open-access and inequality in non-human biological sciences. *Scientometrics*, 124:1663–1675.

Grey, A., Avenell, A., and Bolland, M. (2021). Timeliness and content of retraction notices for publications by a single research group. *Accountability in Research*, 0(0):1–32. https://doi.org/10.1080/08989621.2021.1920409.

Gross, K., and Bergstrom, C.T. (2021). "Why Ex Post Peer Review Encourages High-Risk Research While Ex Ante Review Discourages It." ArXiv:2106.13282 [Physics], June 24, 2021. http://arxiv.org/abs/2106.13282.

Grossmann, A., and Brembs, B. (2021). Current Market Rates for Scholarly Publishing Services. F1000Research. https://doi.org/10.12688/f1000research.27468.2.

Hagan, A. K., Topçuoğlu, B. D., Gregory, M. E., Barton, H. A., and Schloss, P. D. (2020). Women Are Underrepresented and Receive Differential Outcomes at ASM Journals: a Six-Year Retrospective Analysis. *mBio*, 11(6).

Hagve, M. (2020). The money behind academic publishing. *Tidsskrift for Den norske legeforening*.

Hall, N. (2014). The Kardashian index: a measure of discrepant social media profile for scientists. *Genome Biology*, 15(7):424.

Hall, S., Moskovitz, C., and Pemberton, M. (2021). Understanding Text Recycling: A Guide for Researchers. https://textrecycling.org/.

Harington, R. M. (2020). The importance of scholarly societies for research and community support. *FASEB BioAdvances*, 2(9):573–574.

Hartley, J. and Cabanac, G. (2017). The delights, discomforts, and downright furies of the manuscript submission process. *Learned Publishing*, 30(2):167–172.

Haustein, S., Bowman, T. D., and Costas, R. (2015). When is an article actually published? An analysis of online availability, publication, and indexation dates. *arXiv:1505.00796 [cs]*. arXiv: 1505.00796.

Heesen, R. and Bright, L. K. (2020). Is Peer Review a Good Idea? *The British Journal for the Philosophy of Science*, 2019(July):1–31.

Helmer, M., Schottdorf, M., Neef, A., and Battaglia, D. (2017). Gender bias in scholarly peer review. *eLife*, 6:e21718.

Helmer, S., Blumenthal, D. B., and Paschen, K. (2020). What is meaningful research and how should we measure it? *Scientometrics*, 125(1):153–169.

Heneberg, P. (2016). From Excessive Journal Self-Cites to Citation Stacking: Analysis of Journal Self-Citation Kinetics in Search for Journals, Which Boost Their Scientometric Indicators. *PLOS ONE*, 11(4):e0153730.

Hirsch, J. E. (2005). An index to quantify an individual's scientific research output. *Proceedings of the National Academy of Sciences*, 102(46):16569–16572.

Hopewell, S., Witt, C. M., Linde, K., Icke, K., Adedire, O., Kirtley, S., and Altman, D. G. (2018). Influence of peer review on the reporting of primary outcome(s) and statistical analyses of randomised trials. *Trials*, 19(1):30.

Huisman, J. and Smits, J. (2017). Duration and quality of the peer review process: the author's perspective. *Scientometrics*, 113(1):633–650.

Husemann, M., Rogers, R., Meyer, S., and Habel, J. C. (2017). "Publicationism" and scientists' satisfaction depend on gender, career stage and the wider academic system. *Palgrave Communications*, 3(1):1–10.

Hussinger, K. and Pellens, M. (2019). Scientific misconduct and accountability in teams. *PLOS ONE*, 14(5):e0215962.

Hyland, K. and Jiang, F. K. (2020). This work is antithetical to the spirit of research: An anatomy of harsh peer reviews. *Journal of English for Academic Purposes*, 46:100867.

Ioannidis, J. P. A. (2005). Why most published research findings are false. *PLoS Medicine*, 2(8):e124.

Ioannidis, J. P. A. (2008). Measuring Co-Authorship and Networking-Adjusted Scientific Impact. *PLOS ONE*, 3(7):e2778.

Ioannidis, J. P. A., Boyack, K., and Wouters, P. F. (2016). Citation Metrics: A Primer on How (Not) to Normalize. *PLOS Biology*, 14(9):e1002542.

Ioannidis, J. P. A. and Thombs, B. D. (2019). A user's guide to inflated and manipulated impact factors. *European Journal of Clinical Investigation*, 49(9):e13151.

Janicke Hinchliffe, L. (2019). Transformative Agreements: A Primer. https://scholarlykitchen.sspnet.org/2019/04/23/transformative-agreements/.

Janicke Hinchliffe, L. (2021). Explaining the Rights Retention Strategy. https://scholarlykitchen.sspnet.org/2021/02/17/rights-retention-strategy/.

Jefferson, T., Alderson, P., Wager, E., and Davidoff, F. (2002). Effects of editorial peer review: a systematic review. *JAMA*, 287(21):2784–2786.

Jennions, M. D. and Møller, A. P. (2002). Publication bias in ecology and evolution: an empirical assessment using the 'trim and fill' method. *Biological Reviews*, 77(2):211–222.

Jiang, S. (2021). Understanding authors' psychological reactions to peer reviews: a text mining approach. *Scientometrics*, 126:6085–6103. https://doi.org/10.1007/s11192-021-04032-8.

Jinha, A. E. (2010). Article 50 million: an estimate of the number of scholarly articles in existence. *Learned Publishing*, 23(3):258–263.

Kenar, J. A. (2016). Dear Authors: We Do Read Your Cover Letters. *Journal of the American Oil Chemists' Society*, 93(9):1171–1172.

Khoo, S. (2018). There is little evidence to suggest peer reviewer training programmes improve the quality of reviews. https://blogs.lse.ac.uk/impactofsocialsciences/2018/05/23/there-is-little-evidence-to-suggest-peer-reviewer-training-programmes-improve-the-quality-of-reviews/.

Khoo, S. (2019). Article Processing Charge Hyperinflation and Price Insensitivity: An Open Access Sequel to the Serials Crisis. *LIBER Quarterly*, 29(1):1–18.

Khoo, S. (2021). Why the Plan S Rights Retention Strategy Probably Won't Work. https://scholarlykitchen.sspnet.org/2021/07/27/guest-post-why-the-plan-s-rights-retention-strategy-probably-wont-work/.

Kidwell, M. C., Lazarević, L. B., Baranski, E., Hardwicke, T. E., Piechowski, S., Falkenberg, L.-S., Kennett, C., Slowik, A., Sonnleitner, C., Hess-Holden, C., Errington, T. M., Fiedler, S., and Nosek, B. A. (2016). Badges to Acknowledge Open Practices: A Simple, Low-Cost, Effective Method for Increasing Transparency. *PLOS Biology*, 14(5):e1002456.

Koppers, L., Wormer, H., and Ickstadt, K. (2017). Towards a Systematic Screening Tool for Quality Assurance and Semiautomatic Fraud Detection for Images in the Life Sciences. *Science and Engineering Ethics*, 23(4):1113–1128.

Kramer, B., and Bosman, J. (2016). "Innovations in Scholarly Communication - Global Survey on Research Tool Usage." *F1000Research*, https://doi.org/10.12688/f1000research.8414.1.

Kriegeskorte, N., Walther, A., and Deca, D. (2012). An emerging consensus for open evaluation: 18 visions for the future of scientific publishing. *Frontiers in Computational Neuroscience*, 6:94.

Krishna, A. and Soumyaja, D. (2020). Playing safe games–thematic analysis of victims' perspectives on gendered bullying in academia. *Journal of Aggression, Conflict and Peace Research*, 12(4):197–208.

Kun, Ã. (2018). Publish and Who Should Perish: You or Science? *Publications*, 6(2):18.

Kwok, L. S. (2005). The White Bull Effect: Abusive Coauthorship and Publication Parasitism. *Journal of Medical Ethics*, 31(9):554–56. https://doi.org/10.1136/jme.2004.010553.

Larivière, V. and Costas, R. (2016). How Many Is Too Many? On the Relationship between Research Productivity and Impact. *PLOS ONE*, 11(9):e0162709.

Larivière, V., Haustein, S., and Mongeon, P. (2015). Big Publishers, Bigger Profits: How the Scholarly Community Lost the Control of its Journals. *Libraries in Crisis*, 5(2):9.

Larivière, V., Haustein, S., and Mongeon, P. (2015). "The Oligopoly of Academic Publishers in the Digital Era." PLOS ONE 10: e0127502. https://doi.org/10.1371/journal.pone.0127502.

Lee, C. J., Sugimoto, C. R., Zhang, G., and Cronin, B. (2013). Bias in peer review. *Journal of the American Society for Information Science and Technology*, 64(1):2–17.

Link, A. M. (1998). US and Non-US Submissions: An Analysis of Reviewer Bias. *JAMA*, 280(3):246.

Lithgow, G. J., Driscoll, M., and Phillips, P. (2017). A long journey to reproducible results. *Nature*, 548(7668):387–388.

Logan, C. J. (2017). "We Can Shift Academic Culture through Publishing Choices." F1000Research, https://doi.org/10.12688/f1000research.11415.2.

Lund, B. D. and Wang, T. (2020). An Analysis of Spam from Predatory Publications in Library and Information Science. *Journal of Scholarly Publishing*, 52(1):35–45.

Macleod, M., Collings, A. M., Graf, C., Kiermer, V., Mellor, D., Swaminathan, S., Sweet, D., and Vinson, V. (2021). The MDAR (Materials Design Analysis Reporting) Framework for transparent reporting in the life sciences. *Proceedings of the National Academy of Sciences*, 118(17).

Mahmoudi, M. (2020). A survivor's guide to academic bullying. *Nature Human Behaviour*, 4(11):1091–1091.

Mahmoudi, M. and Keashly, L. (2021). Filling the space: a framework for coordinated global actions to diminish academic bullying. *Angewandte Chemie*, 133(7):3378–3384.

Mahoney, M. J. (1977). Publication prejudices: An experimental study of confirmatory bias in the peer review system. *Cognitive Therapy and Research*, 1(2):161–175.

Malaga-Trillo, E. and Gerlach, G. (2004). Meyer case poses a challenge to the system. *Nature*, 431(7008):505–506.

Manlove, K. R. and Belou, R. M. (2018). Authors and editors assort on gender and geography in high-rank ecological publications. *PLOS ONE*, 13(2):e0192481.

Marcus, A. A. (2020). Spider researcher uses legal threats, public records requests to prevent retractions. https://retractionwatch.com/2020/08/20/spider-researcher-uses-legal-threats-public-records-requests-to-halt-correction-of-the-record/.

Marshall, B. M. and Strine, C. T. (2021). Make like a glass frog: In support of increased transparency in herpetology. *Herpetological Journal*, 31(1):35–45.

Martin, B. R. (2016). Editors' JIF-boosting stratagems – Which are appropriate and which not? *Research Policy*, 45(1):1–7.

Martin-Martin, A., Orduna-Malea, E., Thelwall, M., and Lopez-Cozar, E. D. (2018). Google Scholar, Web of Science, and Scopus: A systematic comparison of citations in 252 subject categories. *Journal of informetrics*, 12(4):1160–1177.

Martín-Martín, A., Thelwall, M., Orduna-Malea, E., and Delgado López-Cózar, E. (2021). Google Scholar, Microsoft Academic, Scopus, Dimensions, Web of Science, and OpenCitations' COCI: a multidisciplinary comparison of coverage via citations. *Scientometrics*, 126(1):871–906.

Matheson, A. (2016). Ghostwriting: the importance of definition and its place in contemporary drug marketing. *BMJ*, 354:i4578.

Mayden, K. D. (2012). Peer Review: Publication's Gold Standard. *Journal of the Advanced Practitioner in Oncology*, 3(2):117–122.

McKiernan, E. C., Schimanski, L. A., Muñoz Nieves, C., Matthias, L., Niles, M. T., and Alperin, J. P. (2019). Use of the Journal Impact Factor in academic review, promotion, and tenure evaluations. *eLife*, 8:e47338.

McPeek, M. A., Deangelis, D. L., Shaw, R. G., Moore, A. J., Rausher, M. D., Strong, D. R., Ellison, A. M., Barrett, L., Rieseberg, L., Breed, M. D., Sullivan, J., Osenberg, C. W., Holyoak, M., and Elgar, M. A. (2009). The golden rule of reviewing. *American Naturalist*, 173(5):E155–E158.

Measey, J. (2011). The past, present and future of African herpetology. *African Journal of Herpetology*, 60(2):89–100. https://doi.org/10.1080/21564574.2011.628413.

Measey, J. (2018). Europe's plan S could raise everyone else's publication paywall. *Nature*, 562(7728):494–494. https://www.nature.com/articles/d41586-018-07152-z.

Measey, J. (2021). *How to write a PhD in biological sciences: A guide for the uninitiated*. CRC Press, Boca Raton, Florida. http://www.howtowriteaphd.org/.

Mellor, D., Roettger, T., Schmalz, X., Cashin, A., and Bagg, M. (2019). Advocating for Change in How Science is Conducted to Level the Playing Field. https://youtu.be/3WX0gXXztlE.

Merton, R. K. (1968). The Matthew Effect in Science: The reward and communication systems of science are considered. *Science*, 159(3810):56–63.

Metze, K. (2010). Bureaucrats, researchers, editors, and the impact factor: a vicious circle that is detrimental to science. *Clinics*, 65(10):937–940.

Michael, A. (2021). Wiley Acquires Hindawi: An Interview with Judy Verses and Liz Ferguson. https://scholarlykitchen.sspnet.org/2021/01/11/wiley-acquires-hindawi-interview/.

Mishra, S., Fegley, B. D., Diesner, J., and Torvik, V. I. (2018). Self-citation is the hallmark of productive authors, of any gender. *PLOS ONE*, 13(9):e0195773.

Morales, E. McKiernan, E.C., Niles, M.T., Schimanski, L., and Alperin, J.P. (2021). How Faculty Define Quality, Prestige, and Impact of Academic Journals. PLOS ONE 16: e0257340. https://doi.org/10.1371/journal.pone.0257340.

Mizzaro, S. (2003). Quality Control in Scholarly Publishing: A New Proposal. *Journal of the American Society for Information Science and Technology*, 54:989–1005. https://doi.org/10.1002/asi.10296.

Morgan, R., Hawkins, K., and Lundine, J. (2018). The foundation and consequences of gender bias in grant peer review processes. *CMAJ*, 190(16):E487–E488.

Moustafa, K. (2015). Does the Cover Letter Really Matter? *Science and Engineering Ethics*, 21(4):839–841.

Munafò, M. R., Matheson, I. J., and Flint, J. (2007). Association of the DRD2 gene Taq1A polymorphism and alcoholism: a meta-analysis of case–control studies and evidence of publication bias. *Molecular Psychiatry*, 12(5):454–461.

Munafò, M. R., Nosek, B. A., Bishop, D. V. M., Button, K. S., Chambers, C. D., Percie du Sert, N., Simonsohn, U., Wagenmakers, E.-J., Ware, J. J., and Ioannidis, J. P. A. (2017). A manifesto for reproducible science. *Nature Human Behaviour*, 1(1):1–9.

Nakada, M. and Xu, L. (2018). No Room For New Blood: Harvard's Aging Faculty. https://www.thecrimson.com/article/2018/5/23/yir-aging-faculty/.

Niles, M. T., Schimanski, L.A., McKiernan, E.C., and Alperin, J.P. (2020). Why We Publish Where We Do: Faculty Publishing Values and Their Relationship to Review, Promotion and Tenure Expectations. PLOS ONE 15(3): e0228914. https://doi.org/10.1371/journal.pone.0228914.

Nissen, S.B., Magidson, T., Gross, K., and Bergstrom, C.T. (2016). Publication Bias and the Canonization of False Facts. *ELife* 5: e21451. https://doi.org/10.7554/eLife.21451.

Nosek, B. (2019). Strategy for Culture Change. https://www.cos.io/blog/strategy-for-culture-change.

Nuzzo, R. (2015). How scientists fool themselves – and how they can stop. *Nature*, 526(7572):182–185.

Nuñez, M. A. and Amano, T. (2021). Monolingual searches can limit and bias results in global literature reviews. *Nature Ecology & Evolution*, 5(3):264–264.

O'Carroll, C., Brennan, N., Hyllseth, B., Kohl, U., O'Neill, G., and Van Den Berg, R. (2017). Providing researchers with the skills and competencies they need to practise Open Science: Open Science Skills Working Group Report. Report, European Commission DG-RTG.

Okike, K., Hug, K. T., Kocher, M. S., and Leopold, S. S. (2016). Single-blind vs Double-blind Peer Review in the Setting of Author Prestige. *JAMA*, 316(12):1315.

Oransky, A. I. (2011). The Year of the Retraction: A look back at 2011. https://retractionwatch.com/2011/12/30/the-year-of-the-retraction-a-look-back-at-2011/.

Oransky, A. I. (2021). Elsevier journals ask Retraction Watch to review COVID-19 papers. https://retractionwatch.com/2021/03/09/elsevier-journals-ask-retraction-watch-to-review-covid-19-papers/.

Pannell, D. J. (2002). Prose, Psychopaths and Persistence: Personal Perspectives on Publishing. *Canadian Journal of Agricultural Economics/Revue canadienne d'agroeconomie*, 50(2):101–115.

Parish, A. J., Boyack, K. W., and Ioannidis, J. P. A. (2018). Dynamics of co-authorship and productivity across different fields of scientific research. *PLOS ONE*, 13(1):e0189742.

Parker, T. H., Griffith, S. C., Bronstein, J. L., Fidler, F., Foster, S., Fraser, H., Forstmeier, W., Gurevitch, J., Koricheva, J., Seppelt, R., Tingley, M. W., and Nakagawa, S. (2018). Empowering peer reviewers with a checklist to improve transparency. *Nature Ecology & Evolution*, 2(6):929–935.

Penders, B., and Shaw, D.M. (2020). Civil Disobedience in Scientific Authorship: Resistance and Insubordination in Science. *Accountability in Research 27*, 347–71. https://doi.org/10.1080/08989621.2020.1756787.

Pennisi, E. (2020). Embattled spider biologist seeks to delay additional retractions of problematic papers. *Science*. https://www.sciencemag.org/news/2020/03/embattled-spider-biologist-seeks-delay-additional-retractions-problematic-papers.

Perry, G., Bertoluci, J., Bury, B., Hansen, R. W., Jehle, R., Measey, J., Moon, B. R., Muths, E., and Zuffi, M. A. L. (2012). The 'peer' in 'Peer Review'. *African Journal of Herpetology*, 61(1):1–2. https://doi.org/10.1080/21564574.2012.658665.

Peterson, A. T., Anderson, R. P., Beger, M., Bolliger, J., Brotons, L., Burridge, C. P., Cobos, M. E., Cuervo-Robayo, A. P., Di Minin, E., and Diez, J. (2019). Open access solutions for biodiversity journals: Do not replace one problem with another. *Diversity and Distributions*, 25(1):5–8.

Piller, C. (2021). Disgraced COVID-19 studies are still routinely cited. *Science*, 371(6527):331–332.

Pinfield, S., Salter, J., and Bath, P. A. (2016). The 'total cost of publication' in a hybrid open-access environment: Institutional approaches to funding journal article-processing charges in combination with subscriptions. *Journal of the Association for Information Science and Technology*, 67(7):1751–1766.

Piwowar, H. A., Priem, J., Larivière, V., Alperin, J. P., Matthias, L., Norlander, B., Farley, A., West, J., and Haustein, S. (2018). The state of OA: a large-scale analysis of the prevalence and impact of Open Access articles. *PeerJ*, 6:e4375.

Pooley, Jefferson. "Surveillance Publishing." SocArXiv, November 18, 2021. https://doi.org/10.31235/osf.io/j6ung.

Posada, Alejandro, and George Chen. "Inequality in Knowledge Production: The Integration of Academic Infrastructure by Big Publishers." In ELPUB 2018, https://doi.org/10.4000/proceedings.elpub.2018.30.

Potvin, D. A., Burdfield-Steel, E., Potvin, J. M., and Heap, S. M. (2018). Diversity begets diversity: A global perspective on gender equality in scientific society leadership. *PLOS ONE*, 13(5):e0197280.

Poulson-Ellestad, K., Hotaling, S., Falkenberg, L. J., and Soranno, P. (2020). Illuminating a Black Box of the Peer Review System: Demographics,

Experiences, and Career Benefits of Associate Editors. *Limnology & Oceanography Bulletin*, 29(1):11–17.

Powers, S. M. and Hampton, S. E. (2019). Open science, reproducibility, and transparency in ecology. *Ecological Applications*, 29(1):e01822.

Poynder, R. (2019). *Open access: Could defeat be snatched from the jaws of victory?* Self Published. https://richardpoynder.co.uk/Jaws.pdf.

Poynder, R. (2020). *Information Wants To Be Free v.2*. Self Published. http://archive.org/details/information-wants-to-be-free_20210101.

Priem, J., Groth, P., and Taraborelli, D. (2012). The Altmetrics Collection. *PLOS ONE*, 7(11):e48753.

Quan, W., Chen, B., and Shu, F. (2017). Publish or impoverish: An investigation of the monetary reward system of science in China (1999-2016). *Aslib Journal of Information Management*, 69(5):486–502.

Raff, J. (2013). How to become good at peer review: A guide for young scientists. https://violentmetaphors.com/2013/12/13/how-to-become-good-at-peer-review-a-guide-for-young-scientists/.

Raju, R. and Pietersen, J. (2017). Library as Publisher: From an African Lens. *Journal of Electronic Publishing*, 20(2).

Rennie, D. and Flanagin, A. (1994). Authorship! Authorship!: Guests, Ghosts, Grafters, and the Two-Sided Coin. *JAMA*, 271(6):469–471.

Ritchie, S. (2020). *Science Fictions: How Fraud, Bias, Negligence, and Hype Undermine the Search for Truth*. Metropolitan Books.

Rittel, H. W. J. and Webber, M. M. (1973). Dilemmas in a general theory of planning. *Policy Sciences*, 4(2):155–169.

Rittman, M. (2020). Fast, citable feedback: Peer reviews for preprints and other content types. https://www.crossref.org/blog/fast-citable-feedback-peer-reviews-for-preprints-and-other-content-types/.

Ross-Hellauer, T. (2017). What is open peer review? A systematic review. *F1000Research*, 6:588.

Rothwell, P. M. and Martyn, C. N. (2000). Reproducibility of peer review in clinical neuroscience: Is agreement between reviewers any greater than would be expected by chance alone? *Brain*, 123(9):1964–1969.

Sandström, U. and van den Besselaar, P. (2016). Quantity and/or Quality? The Importance of Publishing Many Papers. *PLOS ONE*, 11(11):e0166149.

Schiltz, M. (2018). Science without publication paywalls: cOAlition S for the realisation of full and immediate Open Access. *PLoS Medicine*, 15(9):e1002663.

Schimel, D., Strong, D. R., Ellison, A. M., Peters, D. P. C., Silver, S., Johnson, E. A., Belnap, J., Classen, A. T., Essington, T. E., Finley, A. O., Inouye, B. D., and Stanley, E. H. (2014). Editors Are Editors, Not Oracles. *The Bulletin of the Ecological Society of America*, 95(4):342–346.

Schroter, S., Black, N., Evans, S., Carpenter, J., Godlee, F., and Smith, R. (2004). Effects of training on quality of peer review: randomised controlled trial. *BMJ*, 328(7441):673.

Sidiropoulos, A., Katsaros, D., and Manolopoulos, Y. (2007). Generalized Hirsch h-index for disclosing latent facts in citation networks. *Scientometrics*, 72(2):253–280.

Silbiger, N. J. and Stubler, A. D. (2019). Unprofessional peer reviews disproportionately harm underrepresented groups in STEM. *PeerJ*, 7:e8247.

Simmons, J. P., Nelson, L. D., and Simonsohn, U. (2011). False-positive psychology: Undisclosed flexibility in data collection and analysis allows presenting anything as significant. *Psychological Science*, 22(11):1359–1366.

Smaldino, P. E. and McElreath, R. (2016). The natural selection of bad science. *Royal Society Open Science*, 3(9):160384.

Smith, E. M. (2021). Reimagining the peer-review system for translational health science journals. *Clinical and Translational Science*. 14:1210–1221

Song, F., Eastwood, A., Gilbody, S., Duley, L., and Sutton, A. (2000). Publication and related biases: a review. *Health Technology Assessment*, 4(10):1–115.

Sánchez-Tójar, A., Nakagawa, S., Sánchez-Fortún, M., Martin, D. A., Ramani, S., Girndt, A., Bókony, V., Kempenaers, B., Liker, A., Westneat, D. F., Burke, T., and Schroeder, J. (2018). Meta-analysis challenges a textbook example of status signalling and demonstrates publication bias. *eLife*, 7:e37385.

Teixeira da Silva, J. A. (2021a). Abuse of ORCID's weaknesses by authors who use paper mills. *Scientometrics*. 126(7):6119–6125

Teixeira da Silva, J. A. (2021b). The Matthew effect impacts science and academic publishing by preferentially amplifying citations, metrics and status. *Scientometrics*, 126(6):5373–5377.

Teixeira da Silva, J. A., Al-Khatib, A., Katavić, V., and Bornemann-Cimenti, H. (2018). Establishing Sensible and Practical Guidelines for Desk Rejections. *Science and Engineering Ethics*, 24(4):1347–1365.

Tennant, J. (2017). The open access citation advantage. *Collection*. https://www.scienceopen.com/collection/OA_cite.

Thurner, S. and Hanel, R. (2011). Peer-review in a world with rational scientists: Toward selection of the average. *The European Physical Journal B*, 84(4):707–711.

Tolsgaard, M. G., Ellaway, R., Woods, N., and Norman, G. (2019). Salami-slicing and plagiarism: How should we respond? *Advances in Health Sciences Education*, 24(1):3–14.

Tomkins, A., Zhang, M., and Heavlin, W. D. (2017). Single versus Double Blind Reviewing at WSDM 2017. *arXiv:1702.00502 [cs]*. arXiv: 1702.00502.

Toro, V. P., Padhye, A. D., Biware, M. V., and Ghaya, N. A. (2019). Retraction Note to: Larvicidal effects of GC-MS fractions from leaf extracts of Cassia uniflora Mill non Spreng. *Journal of Biosciences*, 44(4):76.

Travis, G. and Collins, H. (1991). New Light on Old Boys: Cognitive and Institutional Particularism in the Peer Review System. *Science, Technology, & Human Values*, 16(3):322–341.

Tregenza, T. (2002). Gender bias in the refereeing process? *Trends in Ecology & Evolution*, 17(8):349–350.

Valdez, D., Vorland, C. J., Brown, A. W., Mayo-Wilson, E., Otten, J., Ball, R., Grant, S., Levy, R., Svetina Valdivia, D., and Allison, D. B. (2020). Improving open and rigorous science: ten key future research opportunities related to rigor, reproducibility, and transparency in scientific research. *F1000Research*, 9:1235.

Vale, R. D. (2015). "Accelerating Scientific Publication in Biology. *Proceedings of the National Academy of Sciences* 112:13439–46. https://doi.org/10.1073/pnas.1511912112.

Van Dongen, S. (2011). Associations between asymmetry and human attractiveness: Possible direct effects of asymmetry and signatures of publication bias. *Annals of Human Biology*, 38(3):317–323. https://doi.org/10.3109/03014460.2010.544676.

van Eck, N. J. and Waltman, L. (2010). Software survey: VOSviewer, a computer program for bibliometric mapping. *Scientometrics*, 84(2):523–538.

VanDenBerg, R., Nezami, N., Nguyen, V., Sicklick, J. K., and Weiss, C. R. (2021). A Solution to Academic Radiology's Experience With Solicitation E-mails From Predatory Journals. *American Journal of Roentgenology*, 216(1):233–240.

Van Noorden, R. (2013). "Open Access: The True Cost of Science Publishing." Nature 495(7442):426–29. https://doi.org/10.1038/495426a.

Voelkl, B., Altman, N. S., Forsman, A., Forstmeier, W., Gurevitch, J., Jaric, I., Karp, N. A., Kas, M. J., Schielzeth, H., Van de Casteele, T., and Würbel, H. (2020). Reproducibility of animal research in light of biological variation. *Nature Reviews Neuroscience*, 21(7):384–393.

Vogel, G. (2014). German University Tells Elsevier 'No Deal'. https://www.sciencemag.org/news/2014/03/german-university-tells-elsevier-no-deal.

Wager, E. (2006a). Suspected fabricated data in a submitted manuscript. Technical report, Committee on Publication Ethics. https://doi.org/10.24318/cope.2019.2.3.

Wager, E. (2006b). Suspected ghost, guest or gift authorship. Technical report, Committee on Publication Ethics. https://doi.org/10.24318/cope.2019.2.18.

Wager, E. (2006c). Suspected plagiarism in a submitted manuscript. Technical report, Committee on Publication Ethics. https://publicationethics.org/node/19701.

Wager, E., Singhvi, S., and Kleinert, S. (2015). Too much of a good thing? An observational study of prolific authors. *PeerJ*, 3:e1154.

Wang, P., You, S., Manasa, R., and Wolfram, D. (2016). Open Peer Review in Scientific Publishing: A Web Mining Study of Authors and Reviewers. *Journal of Data and Information Science*, 1(4):60–80.

Williams, C. F. (2021). *Move! The New Science of Body Over Mind*. Profile Books.

Wislar, J. S., Flanagin, A., Fontanarosa, P. B., and DeAngelis, C. D. (2011). Honorary and ghost authorship in high impact biomedical journals: a cross sectional survey. *BMJ*, 343:d6128.

Woolston, C. (2014). Clash over the Kardashians of science. *Nature*, 512(7513):117–117.

Woolston, C. (2016). Faking it. *Nature*, 529(7587):555–557.

Woolston, C. (2019). PhDs: the tortuous truth. *Nature*, 575(7782):403–406.

Xie, Y. (2016). *Bookdown: authoring books and technical documents with R markdown*. CRC Press.

Xie, Y., Allaire, J. J., and Grolemund, G. (2018). *R markdown: The definitive guide*. CRC Press.

Zong, Q., Xie, Y., and Liang, J. (2020). Does open peer review improve citation count? Evidence from a propensity score matching analysis of PeerJ. *Scientometrics*, 125(1):607–623.

Zvereva, E. L. and Kozlov, M. V. (2021). Biases in ecological research: attitudes of scientists and ways of control. *Scientific Reports*, 11(1):226.

Index

Note: Locators in *italics* represent figures and **bold** indicate tables in the text.

Text Printed and Bound by Corcoran and Information privacy contact from
FC representative DJ SK read from https://books.com Tel d r & Dynels
Verlag GmbH Kaulbachstraße 23, 80121 München, Germany.